You Are a Miracle

How To Lose Weight and Love Your Body Too

LIZZIE MERRITT

TABLE OF CONTENTS

INTRODUCTION

I sat at my kitchen table reading another diet book (the 8th? 9th? I forget). This one would be....THE. ONE.

The one that would help me figure out how to get there. How to finally lose the weight and reach my version of "*the after picture.*"

But the words began to blur together. This book wasn't telling me anything new. I'd already read about how hormones impact weight loss in diet book number 4. I already knew which macros to eat in which proportions from diet book number 6.

Finally, I just…stopped.

I looked up.

"This is ridiculous." I thought. "This is insane."

None of these books had anything new to tell me. I had tried all the diets. I exercised regularly. No matter what I saw in the mirror, all I could still see and feel were the things that were not yet right about my body. The harder I worked, the farther I seemed to get from my goal.

That day at my kitchen table I thought, "If diet and exercise aren't getting me to where I want to go, then there has to be something more to this puzzle. What if it is less about what's on my plate, and more about what's between my ears?"

I had no idea how right I was.

I'm assuming if you're reading this then maybe you've felt that way too. Maybe you've been struggling with your weight since elementary school and it's hard to remember a time when you weren't either "on" or "off" a diet. Maybe you put on some weight after college or after your kids were born and tried Whole30 or keto to see if that would "jump start" your weight loss. Maybe you've gained and lost weight several times, but always seem to fall back into old habits.

And maybe, just maybe, you've looked at old pictures of yourself and thought, "Wow, I look so skinny in this picture! I wish I could have that body now." But then you remember how you felt about yourself when that picture was taken. You wanted to lose weight then too.

And you secretly begin to wonder…if you didn't feel great about yourself back then, (when you DID look good!) then what does it REALLY take to feel happy with your body and confident in your skin?

The answer is not found in a diet book. Diets make you feel terrible about yourself because they say, "just follow these simple rules" and you feel like YOU'RE the problem when you know *what* to do, but you can't seem to make yourself do it.

How do diet rules help you when it's 5:37p.m. after a long day when your daughter needs help with her science project, there's a problem with the invoices at work, and you're worried about your mom's recent diagnosis?

Diet books can give you rules to follow, but they don't help you with things like cravings, stress, weekends, and don't even get me started on self-sabotage.

If that weren't bad enough, there's another sneaky secret the diet books don't tell you.

You can reach your "ideal weight" and still not be happy. We THINK that reaching a number on the scale will make us happy. But that's a mirage.

This is not another diet book. Because all diets work...if you can stick to them for the rest of your life.

This book is about the messy stuff. The things that get in the way of those diet rules. If you've ever struggled to follow a program consistently, inexplicably sabotaged yourself, or asked "What the hell is wrong with me?" then this book is for you.

This is a book about what happens between "I'm going on a diet!" and actually getting to a place where you're happy with your body, whether the scale shows that magic number or not.

The strategies in this book give you the opportunity to explore and discover the things that are holding you back and how to overcome them.

It is an invitation to examine what thoughts and beliefs might be at the root of your dissatisfaction, your lack of confidence, and your reluctance to look in the mirror.

Because you have something brilliant to give to the world and every moment you spend feeling "not enough" is a moment that you're not shining as bright as you're meant to.

You are a masterpiece.

A piece of the master.

You are a miracle.

You deserve to feel amazing and beautiful and to recognize how incredible your body is and how magnificent you are. I don't want you to spend one more minute carrying around that 50-pound suitcase of emotional weight that comes with feeling unhappy about yourself and your body. It's time to empty out that suitcase of old shame and heavy thoughts and step into your life fully, without holding back because you're waiting until you lose weight.

This is not a diet book. This is a book about helping you see yourself for the miracle that you are.

My deepest wish for you is to help you create a partnership with your body so that you can approach your weight loss journey from a place of love rather than loathe.

I hope that this book leaves you feeling like maybe it's not your fault that you've struggled before. Maybe there is a way to look at weight loss from a different perspective. And maybe, just maybe, there is a way to feel great about yourself, love your body, and lose weight too.

If you really, truly want to live a life where you feel confident in your own skin, it's time to embrace the mental and emotional aspects of weight loss that are underneath the surface calories in, calories out.

This book teaches you the missing piece of the weight loss puzzle:

The piece between your ears.

PART 1
THE PIECE BETWEEN YOUR EARS

Everything Diets Don't Tell You About Weight Loss

CHAPTER 1
HOW WE GOT HERE

My junior year in high school, I would get up at 5:30 a.m. to ride the vintage Schwinn Airdyne stationary bike while studying AP Civics in an effort to burn extra calories before school. In college, I had no idea how to eat healthy, so I ate mostly bagels and Diet Coke, with Slim Fast for dinner to "save calories." Even though I was an athlete in high school and college, I remember constantly worrying about my weight.

After I finished school, my activity level slowed down and exercise became a chore rather than something I looked forward to. Plus, I didn't know how to eat in a way that supported me, so the weight began to creep on.

Fast forward a few years. I got married to a wonderful man, and we had two sweet kiddos. But I found myself feeling exhausted and guilting myself with *"I should work out"* rather than truly wanting to exercise (or actually doing it.) Plus, life was busy! (Is life ever NOT busy?) I was interested in food that was easy, quick, and crowd pleasing. Not always a recipe for healthy meals.

One day, my friend Lynn invited me to dinner for my birthday. She said, "What are you doing next month? Because I am starting a Stroller Strides franchise and you have to come."

"Uhhhmm, ok," I replied.

Soon the Stroller Strides moms became my friends and my community during a time when my most prevalent thought was, "How exactly do I do this mom thing?"

Several months later, Lynn needed help teaching her classes because she was going on maternity leave. She asked me if I'd be willing to get certified and step in for her. I thought, "Sure! But this is a temporary thing, right?"

Pretty soon, I found that I loved teaching fitness. I was surprised that even as an introvert, I could turn on my "coach" persona and make classes fun and leave people smiling.

But here's the thing:

The more I stood in front of the class, the more I felt like an impostor. Who the heck was I to tell these women how to feel great when I didn't like the way my clothes fit and all I could see in the mirror was the cottage cheese on my thighs?

I was far from comfortable with my body. Why should anyone listen to ME?

I felt like I needed to find some secret so that I could teach it to my classes. Naturally, I assumed the secret was to work out more and eat less.

And that's how I found myself at the kitchen table with another diet book in front of me, with this image in my mind of the perfect after picture that felt forever out of reach.

Though I didn't realize it at the time, that day marked a turning point for me.

I realized that going on a diet to lose weight is like going to the Hotel California. You can check out anytime you like, but you can never leave. (And now that song is in my head. Great.)

I began to ask myself, "What's the whole point of losing weight anyway? What am I really after?"

I realized that I just wanted to feel confident. I wanted to go to the pool with my kids and be present instead of obsessing about how I looked in my swimsuit. I wanted to actually enjoy my life instead of carrying around a cloud of self-conscious thoughts all the time.

So I turned in my room key at the Hotel Diet-fornia and decided to focus on the end result - how I wanted to FEEL.

This book is what I've learned.

Why Is It So Hard to Feel Comfortable in Your Own Skin?

Have you ever seen a baby explore and begin to figure out their world through the miracle of their body? As babies, we spend hours in awe and wonder at our bodies discovering the miracle of fingers, toes, and smiles. We know we are a miracle coming into this world. Babies aren't ashamed to ask for (or demand) what they need. Toddlers aren't afraid to say, "Look at me! I did something awesome! In fact, I'm awesome! Can't you tell?"

However, our survival depends on other people. So we learn to look outside of ourselves for validation. We dim the light of our awesome to fit in with the tribe.

We learn that we are not A-OK as we are.

We get conflicting messages. On the one hand, there is this model of perfection (more on that in a sec) that we see everywhere - magazines, commercials, tv shows. The diet and beauty industries tell us quite clearly that we are NOT enough as we are. But we *could* be, if we only buy their products.

On the other hand, we are taught that it is egotistical, arrogant, and self-centered to appreciate our bodies or (gasp!) believe that we are beautiful. Can you imagine saying out loud in seventh grade *"Yeah, I think I'm beautiful."* Just the thought of it feels cringeworthy.

Who are YOU to think you are beautiful? That is for someone else to tell you. Not for you to decide for yourself.

On top of that, caring for yourself can feel selfish. Many of us have natural energy that is nurturing, caring, and supporting. If we care about ourselves too much, then we are less caring about others. And that's bad.

In summary, here's what we learn:

1. You are not okay as you are.
2. Believing you are beautiful is bad.
3. Take care of others first, and yourself last.

Can you see these scripts anywhere in your head? Do they feel true to you?

Is it any wonder that we struggle with our self-image when we have an underlying program that tells us (1) we are not okay as we are, (2) it is dangerous to think too highly of ourselves, (3) and on top of that we've possibly spent years taking care of others' needs first, and neglecting our bodies in the process?

In order to figure out how to fix this pattern, look into the brain and see just exactly what the heck is going on in there.

How Your Brain Is Like Aaron Rogers

My son's favorite football team is the Green Bay Packers. How a Florida kid ended up loving a team from Wisconsin, I'll never know. Nevertheless, I keep up on the NFL stories so I can have something to talk about with him. During the 2021 season, quarterback Aaron Rogers missed a game because of Covid protocols. Aaron Rogers is an expensive player. He gets paid A LOT of money. However, the way the Green Bay Packers played that day shows exactly why it's worth it to pay him so much money. The team was definitely not the same without him.

In the world of the human body, your brain is kinda like the star quarterback - expensive, but worth it.

The brain is a really big energy drain on the human body. At the same time, it's pretty useful, so there's good reason to keep it around! Just as the quarterback hands the ball to the running back or throws to the receiver, the brain parses out functions into different areas of the brain that take up more or less energy in order to be more efficient. Basically, it's really good at delegating.

The conscious mind (primarily the neocortex) is the evolutionarily younger part of the brain. This is where we make conscious decisions, like "I'm going on a diet!"

The subconscious mind is much older and more primitive. This is the part of the brain that is focused on keeping you alive with things like breathing, digestion, the fight-or-flight response, etc. Folks often refer to this part of the brain as "the lizard brain."

11

(More on that in the section on self-sabotage.) Estimates vary, but experts say that up to about 95% of our decisions and actions are dictated by the subconscious mind.

The brain is constantly looking for patterns to delegate to the subconscious mind so that it can save energy. Those patterns become our habits. When something gets delegated to your lower brain, it's outside of our conscious thought because it's a habit.

Sorta like wi-fi. It's there, but you can't see it. All you're really aware of is the result. The result with wi-fi is streaming the latest Marvel movie. The result with the brain is reaching for M&Ms after dinner.

It is a marvelous gift that our brains can do this. It makes life so much easier that we can delegate patterns and habits to auto-pilot. And, like any double-edged sword, it can really wreck our plans when it comes to losing weight.

The brain doesn't have a filter to sort through what is a positive habit or a negative one. It's simply scanning for patterns. When there's a reward attached to the pattern, the brain thinks this pattern is worth repeating. And presto chango - you've got yourself a habit.

But wait! There's more….

While all that is going on, the subconscious mind is on high alert scanning for any change or anything out of the ordinary.

Why?

Remember, the subconscious mind is the evolutionarily older part of the brain. I mean we're talking primitive here. And back in cave-woman days, different meant BAD. Change meant there was a potential threat to your survival.

[Subconscious mind]

- "There's less food than yesterday. Maybe there's a famine coming. Better conserve fat to make sure we have enough reserves for the famine."
- "Hmmm, those berries are different. They could be good to eat, but Cave Gal Sally keeled over from eating something different last month, so I'm steering clear of whatever these are."
- "Was that a rustle in the grass? It could be just the wind. Or it could be dinner! Or it could be something with big, pointy teeth looking to make me its dinner. I think I'll run away."

The brain evolved to proactively look for what is wrong or different with the environment to protect us from predators or other dangers.

These days, our brains are pretty much the same, but our environments are reaaaaally different (thankfully!).

So let's zoom out, shall we?

1. On the one hand, we've got the brain putting anything with a reward attached to it on autopilot, so we don't have to think about it.
2. But that also means we can't really see it, so it's hard to know what's going on beneath the surface.
3. At the same time, the brain is actively looking for what's wrong and avoiding change like your life depends on it (because that used to be true.)

Imagine the subconscious mind is like a factory with minions inside pumping out habits. The minions never question their orders. They just go through the motions of doing their thing, time after time, day after day.

At the door of the subconscious mind factory is this big, burly bouncer whose job is to make sure no new orders get in, unless it's got a reward attached to it.

Then along comes the good idea fairy who says to the bouncer, "I've got a great idea! Let's go on a diet and eat salad for lunch."

The bouncer says, "I hate change. Your ideas are terrible. And unless you've got a reward attached to that salad, my minions aren't changing your habits one bit."

And we wonder why change is so hard!

Here's the tricky part:

Just like we have habits of action (like M&Ms after dinner) we have habits of thought as well (like "I always start off strong and then fall off the wagon"). When the brain delegates a thought habit track to your subconscious minion factory, it can be hard to break out of it because those thoughts begin to feel really true.

How People Are Like Pups

In 1967, before he became known as "the father of positive psychology," Martin Seligman[1] decided he wanted to study what makes people mentally healthy, rather than only focusing on mental illness.

He did an experiment where he gave a small shock to a dog and paired the shock with the sound of a bell. Over time, the dog learned to react to the bell as if it had been shocked, even after the shock was removed.

---

1   Learned Optimism by Martin Seligman

Next, he put the dog in a crate with a small divider down the middle. The dog could see over the divider and could get over it easily. On one side of the divider, the floor was mildly electrified. The floor on the other side of the divider was not.

As you might imagine, when a dog felt the shock on one side of the divider, it would move and find the area that was safe. (Kinda reminds me of The Floor Is Lava. But I digress.)

Here's the crazy part:

The dogs that had been conditioned to the shock with the bell just laid down and whimpered. They didn't try to find an area of the floor with no shock.

They gave up.

Dogs that had not been pre-conditioned to the shock quickly jumped to the non-electrified side of the crate.

Seligman realized that the dogs had developed "learned helplessness." Over time, he noticed the same patterns in people too. When some people experience persistent failure or a traumatic event, they can develop learned helplessness and convince themselves that nothing will work. So they stop trying.

Have you ever felt that way about trying to lose weight?

You work hard to stay within your calorie budget. You've been "good" all week, but the scale isn't moving. Then you have one night where you go a little overboard and the scale goes up two pounds. It's enough to make anyone want to give up and feel like there's no use in even trying.

In his research, Seligman noticed something strange. Not EVERYONE developed learned helplessness in the face of trauma or failure. Some people actually succeeded and thrived when others learned to stop trying.

What the heck was going on with those weirdos?

As he studied this group of people who flourished in the face of failure, he noticed there was something different about the way they explained the events of their lives to themselves.

Instead of feeling hopeless, these optimistic oddballs created a positive, empowering story around the circumstances in their lives.

Why did failure impact people differently depending on how they explained it to themselves?

Because your brain is like the Matrix. Your reality is flexible, depending on how you decide to view it.

You may be thinking "Okay, hold up. You just lost me there." No worries. Hang with me a sec.

Imagine you're in the subway and a man walks in with his kids. The kids are totally rambunctious and loud, and the man is hardly paying any attention to them. You think "Geeze, can't this guy control his kids or at least be engaged enough to realize they're bothering everyone else here?"

Then he looks up from a daze and says, "Oh I'm sorry. We just came from the hospital. I just lost my wife. Their mother. I don't even know what's going on right now."

Suddenly the meaning of the event you witnessed has changed dramatically. Instead of a thoughtless father who can't be bothered to parent his kids, you see a grieving husband and two children who now have to grow up without their mother.

The event didn't change. The meaning of the event changed, and that impacted how you felt about it. Reality became flexible based on how you chose to view it.

The events of the situation are neutral.

We have thoughts about events to create meaning.

Thoughts lead to feelings and emotions.

Feelings lead to actions and results.

I like to think of this using the acronym S.T.E.A.R. Like you're steering the ship of your life (only not quite spelled the same.) Each thing triggers the next, like a waterfall effect.

S - Situation

T - Thoughts

E - Emotions

A - Actions

R - Results

Our brains are meaning-making machines. Though the events of our lives are neutral, they don't feel neutral because of the story we tell ourselves.

Your brain is always trying to make sense of the world. So it creates a story, an explanation, about what those events mean in order for the world to make sense.

That story feels COM-PLETE-LY true.

But is it?

Just like the story of the father in the subway, your thoughts about the events in your life are just thoughts. That doesn't make them true.

How does this apply to the events in your weight loss journey, and how do you explain them to yourself? When something external triggers you, what do you make that mean? How does the meaning your brain creates end up causing you to suffer and thus want to turn to food to feel better?

For example:

- <u>Situation</u>: I stepped on the scale and it's up two pounds.
- <u>Thought</u>: "This will never work."
- <u>Emotion</u>: Defeated.
- <u>Action</u>: Give up.
- <u>Result</u>: Gain ten more pounds.

- <u>Situation</u>: The scale has gone up and down the same three pounds for a month.
- <u>Thought</u>: "I've wasted time. I'm no closer to where I want to be."
- <u>Emotion</u>: *How does this thought make you feel?*
- <u>Action</u>: *When you feel that way, what actions do you take? What results do you get?*
- <u>Result</u>: *What result do you create from those actions?*

- <u>Situation</u>: I've lost five pounds.
- <u>Thought</u>: "I should be further along by now."
- <u>Emotion</u>: *How does this thought make you feel?*
- <u>Action</u>: *When you feel that way, what actions do you take? What results do you get?*
- <u>Result</u>: *What result do you create from those actions?*

- <u>Situation</u>: It's Friday night.
- <u>Thought</u>: "I deserve a break."

- <u>Emotion</u>: *How does this thought make you feel?*
- <u>Action</u>: *When you feel that way, what actions do you take? What results do you get?*
- <u>Result</u>: *What result do you create from those actions?*

You can see how the story you tell yourself about your weight loss efforts makes such a difference. But not all stories are created equal. There's one story that trumps all the rest and is the single biggest factor that can derail your progress.

> *"The mind is its own place. And in itself can make*
> *a Heaven of hell and hell of Heaven."*
> ~*John Milton*

The Shame Spiral of Doom

When I was in seventh grade, I told a lie.

You see, I really wanted to see the movie *Dirty Dancing*. But it was rated PG-13 and I wasn't yet thirteen. Instead of asking if my mom would trust me to see a movie that was rated PG-13 when I was 12, I just assumed she'd say no.

So I lied.

I told her that my friend and I were going to see the movie *North Shore* about a kid from Arizona that moves to Hawaii to surf.

The whole time I was in the theater I felt like my mom could see me doing something wrong.

When I got home, she asked me about the movie.

"It was good." I said vaguely.

"Tell me about it." she said.

(Oh no. Uhhh, make up something quick.)

"Ummm, well there was this guy....and he goes surfing....and...yeah." (Meanwhile all I could think about was Patrick Swayze and his tight black shirt. What? I was 12.)

Fortunately, mom didn't press me too hard. But I could tell that pretty soon, one lie was gonna lead to another in order to cover up the first lie. I could feel myself getting caught and sucked into a whirlpool of lies stacking on top of one another.

Shame can be like that. It pulls you into this downward spiral that builds on itself until pretty soon you find yourself looking up from the bottom of a bag of Doritos wondering "How did that happen?"

Lemme explain.

The brain is a pretty straightforward machine. It has one main job: keep you alive. One of the main rules the brain follows for ensuring survival is: seek pleasure and avoid pain.

Here's the problem:

When we feel some kind of negative emotion (hurt, pain, stress, boredom) the brain looks for something that will soothe the difficult feeling. Sitting and being present with a difficult emotion feels no bueno. So instead of feeling the feels, your brain looks for something that will relieve the tension of that emotion.

Foods high in sugar, salt, and fat light up the pleasure centers in the brain like a Christmas tree. So from the brain's point of view, food is a quick and reliable way to feel better.

It's a simple equation:

- Problem: Feel bad.
- Solution: Seek to feel better.

- How: Sugar, salt, fat.

However, food is a temporary fix, and it doesn't solve the original issue of whatever difficult emotion you were feeling. So now you're left with the painful emotion that didn't get resolved AND an empty bag of chips.

When we layer in the diet story on top of that, things get really interesting.

Diets purposefully try and make weight loss SEEM simple. "Just follow these simple steps and you'll lose weight."

However, there is so much more going on beneath the surface of the "simple rules" that diets never address. Trying to follow the rules of a diet is like someone telling the captain of the Titanic, "Yeah, just avoid any ice you see on the surface, and you'll be fine."

If it's so simple, why is it so HARD?

Then shame walks into the party and says, "If these rules are so simple, then I must be an idiot because I can't stick to them." It's not a big leap for your brain to jump from the neutral event of eating chips and make it mean…

- I'm fat.
- I have no self-control.
- Why did I eat so much?
- I always do this.
- I'll never be able to lose weight.
- I'm letting myself and everyone else down.
- And so on.

**Original Painful Emotion + I ate too much =
Now I feel even worse**

Our brains take an action and turn it into a meaning. A bag of chips suddenly becomes evidence of my failure as a human being. Shame takes that one event and turns it into a weapon I use against myself.

- <u>Situation</u>: I ate chips.
- <u>Thought</u>: "What is wrong with me? Why can't I just do what the diet says? I have no self-control."
- <u>Emotion</u>: Shame, remorse, defeated.
- <u>Action</u>: Eat whatever I want for the rest of the weekend because it's not working anyway.
- <u>Result</u>: Undo all the progress you made last week over a single weekend.

So what started as a simple negative emotion has now become this massive shame show, leaving you stuck at the bottom of the whirlpool feeling like you're doomed.

And on it goes.

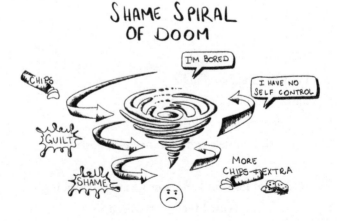

We seem to think that making ourselves feel really bad is the key to making change happen. But it's not true. If you're telling yourself the same old shame story as you're losing weight, then you'll keep getting the same result of going up and down the scale and never feeling happy, no matter what the number says.

Thoughts directly impact results.

Your thinking is the gas that fuels your journey up or down the scale.

The fuel you use to change your life determines what your destination will look like when you get there. Toxic fuel is not sustainable. I never heard a successful, happy person say, "*I just kept beating myself up until I reached long term success.*"

Shame and loathing are the kinds of fuel that lead you to a desolate and empty destination. We need to learn new patterns of thinking and overwrite the old programs that have us stuck in the Shame Spiral of Doom.

If you want a different result, you gotta start where the process begins - with different thoughts.

The power of loving yourself NOW, as you're losing weight, is a superpower.

- I love myself enough to figure this out.
- I love myself even when I make mistakes or fall off the wagon.
- I love myself enough to look for progress rather than perfection.

Choosing your thoughts is not about lying to yourself or turning a blind eye when things are kinda sucky. Honoring all your feelings is really important. Choosing your thoughts on purpose

DOES help you perceive reality in an empowering way that sets you up to take positive action toward the results you want.

The thoughts you have about your weight loss efforts aren't just important. They are EVERYTHING. Your thoughts are the difference between success and failure. Between progress and giving up. Between helplessness and hopefulness.

When you choose your thoughts, new thoughts turn into new actions. New actions turn into new results. Results always start with a thought.

It's time to tell yourself a new story. What have you got to lose?

Start from love and you'll see REAL transformation.

> *"We change by feeling good, not by feeling bad."*
> ~B.J. Fogg

Speaking of thoughts, let's dive right in and talk about the thoughts you have the most often: The ones about yourself.

CHAPTER 2
HOW TO FEEL ENOUGH

"I'm sorry Lizzie. We're going to have to let you go."
WAIT, WHAT?

I'm getting FIRED?

This is not something that happens to ME. I'm the girl that gets straight As and makes the teacher proud. How can I possibly be getting let GO?

I had spent the last six months working in a role that was definitely not a good fit. I was hustling and hustling and instead of feedback, I got *"Yeah, we're gonna give this project to someone else."*

I desperately wanted to hear, *"Hey, good job on this proposal."* Or even, *"I know you worked really hard on this, but here's where it needs work."* Instead, each day at work was like hitting a hot nerve of "I am not enough."

It felt like I was stranded in the Desert of Not Enough. Parched and dehydrated and desperately hustling for a drop of validation.

Strangely, by slamming the door on my ego (ouch), getting fired actually forced me to look for validation in the one place I hadn't considered:

WITHIN MYSELF

I was talking to my friend Gena about it and she said something so wise.

She said *"Lizzie, we can talk about this specific situation and help you get through it. However, the Universe is putting this before you for a reason. If you're constantly looking for your validation and "enoughness" outside of yourself, then once you get through this, you'll keep encountering different versions of this same situation.*

Until.....you can learn to find your worth and "enoughness" within you. THAT'S the lesson that the Universe is inviting you to take on right now.

Do you want to just get over this for now? Or do you want to learn to find your worth within yourself so you can learn this lesson and move on?"

That comment hit me smack in the face.

It's human nature to look for approval and validation outside of ourselves. We learn it when we are young because our survival literally depends on others taking care of us and liking us enough to keep us around. So we learn early to be on the lookout for clues to tell us if the grown-ups are happy or upset with us.

As we grow, we begin to broaden the sphere of people whose opinions we care about. The teacher, our friends, social media likes, the amorphous "they." "What will THEY think?"

Remember, your brain's main job is to keep you alive. Your subconscious mind wants to protect you from being ostracized from the tribe because social death meant literal death if the tribe left you behind. Over time, humans developed an internal navigation system to stay within the good graces of the tribe: The Inner Critic.

It can be so difficult to love yourself and your body when your innate human need to fit in tells you every day that you don't look like you're "supposed" to. It's hard to fit in when you're constantly reminded by the media, mom's expectations, and your own ideas of how you are not enough.

While the Inner Critic is just trying to keep you safe, it can get a little over-zealous sometimes.

The Problem with Self Criticism

I was home for winter break in 1994 when the movie *True Lies*[2] with Arnold Schwarzeneger and Jamie Lee Curtis was a hit at the theaters. Even then I thought this scene was funny.

Helen (played by Jamie Lee):

"How'd it go at the convention? Did you make all the other salesmen jealous?"

Harry (imagine this in Arnold's signature voice):

"It was fantastic! You wouldn't believe it. You should have been there. We were the big hit of the show. With that new model ordering system, the 680 I told you about...I can write up an order and immediately as soon as the customer's name comes up, you see what his credit

---

2   True Lies, 1994 20th Century Fox

line is, what he has ordered in the past, what discount he has gotten…
Every little detail."

Helen:

[Seems bored.] *"Sounds great."*

Harry:

"It was fantastic! That's why I LOVE the computer business."

Helen:

"Listen, the plumber called. He says he has to dig under the slab or
something and that it's gonna cost $600."

Harry:

[Clearly not listening] *"That's okay."*

Helen:

[Stunned] *"It's not okay. It's extortion."*

Harry:

[Barely attentive] *"What did you tell him?"*

Helen:

"I slept with him, and he said he'd knock off $100."

Harry:

[Distracted] *"That's good thinking."*
[Air kisses Helen on the cheek.]
"Bye, honey."

Helen:

[Speechless. Belatedly air kisses back.]

Wait. What did she say? How did he not react to that!?!

The voice in your head can be like that. Chatting away in the background when you're focused on other things. It can be saying all sorts of crazy nonsense and you barely even register what it's saying.

You're so used to it that you're hardly even aware it's there.

And that's a problem because a lot of times, it's not very nice.

If you don't know what you're saying to yourself, you can't change it.

When you look in the mirror, what do you say to yourself? What thoughts go through your head? It doesn't feel very good to have someone constantly pointing out your flaws.

Especially when that someone is always in your head.

Diet culture teaches us to avoid mistakes. We're not taught what to do after we make them. We're not taught how to keep going and not quit after we mess up.

How does hating on yourself help you get any closer to your goal? You can't beat yourself into a better decision tomorrow. It simply doesn't work that way.

Losing weight is so much more about what you tell yourself than about what you put in your mouth.

The thoughts and feelings we have come with a pharmacy. Positive thoughts and feelings trigger the release of dopamine and serotonin, while stress and negative feelings trigger cortisol, which causes inflammation.

Our cells develop more receptors for the chemicals that are more prevalent. So when you get down on yourself or beat yourself up, that triggers cortisol in the body. More cortisol increases inflammation and reduces the body's ability to let go of extra weight.

Because of the Shame Spiral of Doom, we know that feeling bad leads to eating junk food to feel better. Making yourself feel bad about your progress with negative self-talk triggers that downward spiral in your brain.

"For as he thinks in his heart, so he IS."
~Proverbs 23:7

What's the ONE difference between someone who succeeds at long-term weight loss and someone who does not?
- It's NOT the number of times they have a setback.
- It's NOT how perfectly they stick to their plan.

⇒ It is how they talk to themselves.

The person who succeeds keeps going. Even when they fall off the wagon. Even when they screw up their plan. They talk to themselves in a way that allows them to pick themselves up, offer themselves some compassion (not shame and guilt) and keep going.

Learning to forgive yourself is such an important skill for weight loss. Tell yourself at the end of the day, "I love myself. No matter how today went, I am always learning. I want to be the kind of person that can make mistakes and still love myself anyway."

The way you talk to yourself makes a huge difference on how successful you feel. Feeling successful is like Miracle Grow for new habits. It's the magic sauce that helps you keep going long enough for them to stick.

The hardest things about weight loss are not the things we do. It is the things that we think. Learning to direct your thoughts and your brain is the key to weight loss.

"For some reason we are truly convinced that if we criticize ourselves, the criticism will lead to change. If we are harsh, we believe we will end up being kind. If we shame ourselves, we believe we will end up loving ourselves. It has never been true. Not for a moment, that shame leads to love. Only love leads to love."
~Geneen Roth

How To Change the Channel

The good news is that you get to change the channel. Just because you've been thinking a thought your whole life doesn't make it true. The Earth used to be flat....until it wasn't.

The first step to losing weight is being kind to yourself. And the first step to being kind to yourself starts with how you talk to yourself. Changing your self-talk has a multiplier effect because we carry self-talk with us every second of our lives.

Everything you want is on the other side of new actions. And new actions start with new thoughts.

When you criticize yourself, the inner voice asks, "Am I good enough?"

When you offer yourself some self-compassion, that opens you up to ask, "What's good for me?"

Self-compassion defuses the pain of guilt and shame and gives you the grace to be human. By being kind to yourself, you give yourself the chance to get up, dust yourself off, learn, and try again.

The way to "do" self-compassion is pretty straightforward: You treat yourself the same way you'd treat a close friend.

Imagine you met your best friend for coffee, and she confessed how terrible she feels after "blowing her diet" last night. Would you tell her, "I can't believe you ate that! You'll never lose weight."

Probably not.

How might you look at the next slip up or diet mistake as an opportunity to show yourself some compassion instead of judgment?

What about the next time you step on the scale, and you don't like what it says? How can you remind yourself that everyone goes through ups and downs like this?

You're not alone and you're not broken.

> *"Above all else, guard your heart,*
> *for everything you do flows from it."*
> *Proverbs 4:23*

There is a popular Native American legend of a grandfather talking to his grandson and describing the conflict he feels within himself.

Here's one version of it:

The elder was talking to a young warrior one day.

"We have two wolves inside of us. One wolf fights for your happiness. He fiercely defends what you love and leads you to success.

The second wolf fights for your misery. He fiercely defends the things that hurt you and lead to your defeat."

The young warrior asked, "Which wolf wins?"

The elder said "The one you feed."

You can go to work feeding the wolf that says "Losing weight is hard. It never works for me. And I hate exercise too."

Or you can get to work nurturing the wolf that looks for some evidence of progress. You can look for little ways that you are taking better care of yourself 1% at a time. You can choose to look for what's right with you when you look in the mirror.

Listen, you're gonna make mistakes! You're gonna have negative thoughts about yourself sometimes. That's okay! Just give the positive thoughts at least the same amount of airtime in your brain to give yourself a chance. Let the love in!

TAKE IT FURTHER

For a special bonus exercise on self-compassion, go to https://confidentbody.coach/book/ to download this and other bonuses.

We are innately wired to want love and acceptance. It is embedded in our DNA as social animals. And yet when we deny ourselves that same love and acceptance of our bodies, we don't allow ourselves to fully show up in the rest of our lives or relationships.

Loving your body is not a place where you arrive at and it's certainly not a number on the scale. It is a practice. A nurturing.

A daily action. A moment-by-moment choice. Practicing loving your body requires learning to practice self-compassion when you make mistakes and overeat. It requires treating mistakes as invitations to learn and be curious about your own patterns and triggers. It requires proactively choosing what to focus on and where to place your worthiness.

Cultivating self-acceptance and self-love for sustainable weight loss is not a nice-to-have or fluffy. It's not optional. It's a MUST.

Chasing the Horizon

Jennifer and I were on a coaching call and she said, "I saw an old picture of myself yesterday. It was from a trip we took about ten years ago. I saw how skinny I was then, and it made me sad to feel how much weight I've gained. But you know what's crazy? I remember that trip and I remember feeling like I looked fat in my swimsuit. These days, I'd love to have that body back! But even then, I wasn't happy with how I looked."

Jennifer's pictures were photographic evidence proving it's not the size of your body that makes you happy.

In the book *The Happiness Advantage,*[3] Harvard professor Shawn Achor talks about how when we set goals for ourselves, and we often put our happiness "out there" with the finish line.

"I'll be happy when I....[lose weight]."

The trouble with that is we train our brains to learn that happiness is always "out there" and never "here". When we DO reach

---

3   The Happiness Advantage by Shawn Achor

that finish line, it doesn't feel as great as we thought. So we move the target.

"Our goal posts of success keep getting pushed further and further out
so that happiness gets pushed over the horizon."
~Shawn Achor

Just like Jennifer looking at pictures of herself, feeling happy with your body becomes like chasing the horizon...always just out of reach.

Studies show women have negative thoughts about their body up to sixty times a day. That's a lot of thoughts that are actively bringing you down!

Having a negative body image creates a lot of mental and emotional drag in your life. Imagine what you could do with all that energy you're spending on negative body image if you could free yourself from those negative thoughts! I've had clients tell me that they feel so much lighter mentally after our work together simply because they're no longer dragging around so much mental baggage beating themselves down all the time.

Having a healthy body image is not vain, shallow, or no big deal.

- A bad body image keeps you playing small.
  - Denise wanted to apply for a job but worried that no one would listen to her because her size meant "she had no self-discipline."
- It holds you back from going for the things that you want.

- ○ Melanie wanted to start a YouTube channel for her business, but she was afraid what people would think of her size.
- It can impact relationships by preventing you from showing up fully and enjoying everything you can in partnership with another person.
  - ○ Angie was in a loving relationship but held herself back from her partner because she felt "puffy."

Your desire to lose weight is independent of you choosing to love yourself. Any time you tell yourself "I'll be happy when…[I lose 15 lbs]" that means that you're waiting to live your life when you can bring your full light to the world right now.

If you ever want to be happy with your weight, you need to practice being happy "here" (wherever that is) so that your brain doesn't learn to always view happiness as "out there".

What if instead of telling yourself "I'll be happy when I lose weight" you could tell yourself "I'll be happy WHILE I lose weight."

You don't need to achieve your goal to feel worthy. You need to feel worthy in order to achieve your goal.

"Success is not the key to happiness. Happiness is the key to success."
~Albert Schweitzer

Choose Your Own Adventure

Did you ever read those *Choose Your Own Adventure* books as a kid? I always loved them because I could imagine the story ending in different ways. (Of course, I always orchestrated it so that it had a happy ending.)

Let's do a Choose Your Own Adventure thought experiment. Except we'll start with alternate beginnings. Wanna play? Here we go.

Imagine this scene:

You're walking down the street on your way to Starbucks. As you walk in, someone is walking out, and they hold the door for you. You thank them and walk by.

What does this person see when they look at you?

Now stop.

Rewind the movie in your mind. Go back to when you got up this morning.

Alternate beginning A:

You woke up this morning and looked in the mirror. The inner critic voice is running rampant, and you see all the things that are wrong with you.

"Ugh. I can't wear sleeveless shirts because my arms are flabby. My rear end looks huge in these pants. My waistband feels tight."

You don't even notice these thoughts playing in your head as you're going through the day. Yet they come along with you everywhere you go.

Later in the day you're walking into Starbucks, and you pass the stranger.

What does this person see?

Alternate beginning B:

You woke up this morning and looked in the mirror. Those inner critic thoughts came up, but you decided to proactively manage your brain instead.

You know that just because thoughts are there doesn't mean they're true nor does it mean you have to believe them.

In this version of reality, you look in the mirror and think "Yeah, okay, these pants don't fit as well as they used to. You know what? I'm going to change into an outfit that I feel great in. Because I deserve to feel awesome in my clothes."

After you change your clothes, you take a moment to intentionally practice appreciating yourself.

"I really like my hair. It's always been one of my favorite features. And my thighs may be bigger than I'd like, but I really appreciate my legs because they are my ticket to anywhere I want to go in this world. I appreciate my eyes because I can see well and there are a lot of things worth seeing today. And I'm working hard at taking care of myself every day. I may not be perfect, but I am worthy."

Those are the thoughts that you're proactively practicing in your mind, and they get to ride along to wherever you're going.

Later in the day you walk into Starbucks, and you pass a stranger.

What does that person see?

Spoiler:

The stranger sees the exact same person in both cases.

You look the same to someone on the street whether you're telling yourself garbage or you're telling yourself how hot you are.

The difference only matters to YOU.

(Though one could argue that you'd hold yourself a lot higher and exude a better energy with the positive thoughts!) The power is in how you feel about yourself vs what someone else thinks of you.

Our brains want to keep believing what they've always believed because those beliefs kept us alive up until this point. ("Why fix it if it isn't broke?") However, while the subconscious mind doesn't see a problem, broken beliefs lead to unfulfilled lives.

Here's the thing about beliefs: You don't have to keep on thinking things that don't serve you. You can think whatever you want.

If you look the same on the outside to a stranger at Starbucks (or to your spouse or your kids or your mother or the moms at preschool drop-off) no matter what story is going on in your brain, why not walk around thinking you're amazing? Your thoughts about yourself don't change how you look on the outside, but they make a HUGE difference to how you experience the world.

If the difference on the outside is minimal, why not CHOOSE to feel good?

Why not?

You may say "Well, because it's a fantasy. I know that I don't *actually* look good. Telling myself I look good would just be a lie."

A) Okay, really?

Think about someone you know who is a larger size, but you think she's amazing and beautiful. I bet you can find an example. (Oprah comes to mind.)

Looking good is not about size. Feeling good is DEFI-NITELY not about size. It's about the thoughts you choose.

B) You already believe things that possibly are not true.

How do you know that you'll be alive tomorrow? Can you prove it? You have no idea if you could die tomorrow, but you choose to believe you'll live because that helps you function. You choose to live with the belief that your life will go on through tomorrow because that belief serves you.

You can choose to believe whatever you want, and nobody can tell you that you can't. Why not choose the thoughts and beliefs that serve you?

C) So what if it IS a fantasy?

Your experience of life is your perception of it. Not reality. You can believe what you want about yourself, and you don't have to justify it.

You can choose to think you're amazing. Or you can think that you have no self-control, or it's dangerous to shine too bright, or you're "less than".

A lot of people choose that. And a lot of them will say, "Well I don't want to be delusional about myself." Really? You'd rather you just think you're "less than" all the time? Which thought is more delusional? And by the way, who gets to decide?

How is choosing to believe the negative thoughts about yourself still serving you? Your brain is a pretty efficient place. If a thought has no use at all, your brain isn't going to keep it around.

So there's likely SOME way that those negative thoughts about yourself serve you.

- Do they reinforce your identity or self-concept? Maybe you've never questioned them before.
- Is it safer to feel small or unseen? Maybe you're less threatening to others if you don't shine as bright as you can.
- Are you following an old script that you learned when you were small? Maybe you're afraid you'll appear boastful or prideful to others (and thus risk rejection from the tribe).
- Is it just easier to believe the negative thoughts about yourself because if you believed you were capable of more, then you'd have to hold yourself to a higher standard?

Give yourself the gift of looking deeper. How do negative thoughts serve you? Question whether or not you want to keep that limiting story. You can't change something if you're not aware of it.

It is your job to manage your brain because left to its own devices, your brain will find everything that's wrong with you. That's the brain's default setting (thank you evolution.)

Managing your brain can and should be part of your daily routine. Just like brushing your hair or taking a shower. It's natural for your hair to get messy and your body to get stinky. So you make a proactive effort to brush your hair and clean your body.

Treat your thoughts the same way! Air those suckers out and let 'em dry!

You get to decide what you're going to think. All of the time. You get to choose what thoughts you focus on.

Just like it's natural for your pupils to constrict when you walk out into the sun or dilate when you go into the dark, it is completely natural for your inner critic to send up negative thoughts meant to protect you. That's okay and it's completely normal.

And just like you can choose to put on your rose tinted sunglasses in the bright sunlight, you can choose to look for what is right with you rather than what is wrong with you. Knowing that is FREEDOM. So why not stack the deck in your favor?

Why not?

> *"To be beautiful means to be yourself.*
> *You don't need to be accepted by others.*
> *You need to accept yourself.*
> *~Thich Nhat Hanh*

Sticks and Stones

"You've been taking My name in vain."

"What? I wouldn't, God!"[4]

Nika was praying for guidance. She was more than a little confused to hear this message from God. Nika always spoke of God in a way to praise Him. She proactively avoided saying "Oh my God" in conversation. She wouldn't even write "OMG" in a text.

"My name is I AM."

---

4 Hunting For Hope by Nika Maples

42

Suddenly Nika was flooded with thoughts of all the times she'd used the phrase "I am…"

I am stupid.

I am a failure.

I am hopeless.

I am fat.

I am ugly.

I am an idiot.

What if the phrase "I am" was holy? What if it were a prayer, honoring what the Divine has created in you? How would that change the words you say after "I am"?

You are a unique and intentional creation.

If God were the sun, then you are a ray of light.

Sticks and stones can break our bones, but words speak right to the heart.

Words matter. Especially the ones that follow "I am…"

I am worthy.

I am beautiful.

I am beloved.

I am enough.

God said to Moses, "I am who I am.
This is what you are to say to the Israelites: 'I am has sent me to you.'"
Exodus 3:14

"I am the Lord; that is my name!"
Isaiah 42:8

Where To Find Enough

There's a Sioux legend[5] about the creation of the Earth and humans.

> The Creator had formed the Earth and the animals and was in the process of conceiving mankind. The Creator said, "I want to hide something from humans until they are ready for it."
>
> The animals asked, "What do you want to hide?"
>
> "The fact that they can create their own reality," the Creator replied.
>
> Ever helpful, the animals volunteered ideas.
>
> "Give it to me," the Eagle said. "And I will hide it on the moon."
>
> "No. One day they will go there and find it," the Creator replied.
>
> The salmon suggested she take it and hide it at the bottom of the ocean. The Creator smiled and said, "No. They will find it there too."
>
> "I will bury it deep within the great plains," said the mighty buffalo. The Creator replied sadly, "No my friend. They will cut the skin of the earth and see it within."
>
> Then a soft voice spoke up. "Put it inside their hearts." It was Grandmother Mole, who could not see with physical eyes, but sees with spiritual wisdom.
>
> The Creator could feel the wisdom of Grandmother Mole's suggestion and said, "It is done."

---

5   Sioux Creation Story https://nativeamericancreationmythology.weebly.com/sioux-creation-myth.html

We've grown up in a culture that is always hustling. We've been taught to go on this external hunt to look for something outside ourselves to feel worthy, to feel enough, to feel better.

Sometimes losing weight can feel like the doorway to our worthiness.

It feels true.

But beliefs are just thoughts we've repeated over and over. And thoughts are just sentences in our minds.

That doesn't make them true.

What if you were taught something that isn't true?

What if your worthiness, your "enoughness", is already there? It's not outside you or something to strive for.

You already have it.

You already ARE it.

Your challenge is simply to receive it.

Your quest is to accept that you are enough.

Your worthiness is like the sun. It always shines. It just seems like it comes and goes from our perspective here on Earth. But it's always there. You can choose to turn away from it or turn toward it and soak it in. But it's always there.

You have the power to create your own reality.

If you want to lose weight, great! But don't do it to find your worthiness.

It's not there.

It's inside you.

"You will never feel okay by way of external accomplishments. Enough comes from the inside....From seeing what you already have, what you've always had."
Ryan Holiday

CHAPTER 3
HOW TO LOVE THE ONE YOU'RE WITH

Perfection Is Not a Thing

"*I want to try this at-home workout program called P90X. And I think we should do it together.*"

I'm sorry, what did you say?

It was the summer of 2009. We had a two-year-old and a four-month-old and my husband had heard about this crazy workout program while he was on deployment the previous spring.

"*Yeah. I saw guys doing these workouts on the ship and they were getting into really good shape.*" He pulled up the infomercial and we watched it together.

Uhm, no.

Hard pass.

Have fun with that.

So he got the program and did workout day #1 on his own. "*This is amazing! I really think it'd be great to do it together.*" Well, he must have missed his calling as a salesman because he talked me into it.

That program was a BEAST. But we committed to show up every morning for 90 days before the kids got up and we did the workouts the best we could. I vividly remember thinking I'd be sore for the rest of my life.

The main thing that intrigued me about the program was the "before and after" pictures. Wow. I still had plenty of baby weight to lose and I was impressed by the transformations of the people in the promo materials.

After we finished the 90 days, I didn't feel like I was "done." I had more weight to lose. So we did another program.

And another.

Over time, a funny thing happened on the way to my after picture.

I never got there.

Oh, I took the pictures. But no matter how I looked, it was never enough. I kept wondering, "When do I arrive? When do I get to say I made it?"

It took me a long time to learn that the after picture is a mirage.

I'm not even talking about how Photoshop can create a picture of someone that looks perfect in the picture when that's not what they actually look like.

What I mean is:

Perfection. Is. Not. A. Thing.

If I said to you, "You need to strive to be ten feet tall. Ten feet tall is the definition of beauty and success for you." What would you think?

A client of mine put it beautifully when she laughed and said, "I would take no personal responsibility for that." Because that's just not something the human body does.

Striving for perfection or the after picture is like asking yourself to be ten feet tall. There will ALWAYS be something you can find that is wrong with you if you are looking for it. Your toes are too big, your ears are too small, and we're not even gonna talk about your tummy or your thighs or your hips.

Perfection is not something that is actually attainable. Which means striving for it is an effort in futility.

My friend, realizing this is FREEDOM.

If you can release yourself from striving for something that is impossible, what a relief it is to be imperfect!!!! You will always be imperfect! Gloriously, uniquely, fabulously imperfect. What a gift to release yourself from the tyranny of striving for whatever your definition of perfection is.

This isn't about ignoring your flaws or pretending they aren't there. Rather, embrace them as friends, as gifts, as part of the uniqueness that is you.

The Japanese understand the concept of admiring and delighting in that which is beautifully imperfect. The phrase

"*wabi-sabi*" means to appreciate beauty that is "imperfect, imper-
manent, and incomplete" in nature.[6]

There are so many things in nature that catch our eye BE-
CAUSE they are unusual and imperfect in some way. Like a piece
of driftwood on the beach or a flower with a petal at a different
angle. Your body will always be wonderfully and beautifully imperfect.

Whatever you're looking for in life, you'll find it.

Perfectionist thinking says, "I have to be winning at weight loss
every minute of the day or I might as well give up. I have to eat
perfectly, or I blew it."

That's like saying you'd rather get a zero on the test than a B-.

What kind of logic is that? How is losing ten pounds instead
of fifteen pounds a failure? How is taking better care of yourself,
even a little bit, a failure?

I've seen women lose 10 pounds but feel miserable because
they're not losing weight fast enough. That thinking leads to
frustration. So they give up and end up gaining twenty pounds.

Let's say you were trying to learn how to play a specific song
on the piano. How many times would you practice it?

A lot, right?

What would you do when you hit the wrong key? What story
would you tell yourself about that little slip up? Would that be
evidence that you'll never figure out how to play this song? Or
would that be information telling you how to improve?

---

6   Wabi-Sabi: The Japanese Philosophy of Embracing Imperfectionism

Weight loss is the same way.

Striving for perfection leads to the bottom of a tub of ice cream.

Embracing imperfection leads to learning, progress, and improvement over time.

Letting go of perfection allows you to make mistakes. It allows you to learn and grow. Letting go of perfection is essential to your success.

Be willing to be imperfect.

"But wait, what's the difference between wanting to get healthy, feel good, and like the way you look versus perfectionism?"

Healthy striving is asking yourself "How can I improve?"

When you're worried, "What will they think?" you're focusing on perfection. Looking for approval and validation outside of yourself leads to perfectionism.

Perfectionism self-talk sounds like: "I hate my clothes. I'm fat and undisciplined. I have no willpower. I need to lose weight in order to accept myself."

Healthy striving self-talk sounds like: "I want to feel healthy and be able to play with my kids. The scale doesn't tell me how I feel, nor does it determine my worth. I want to figure this out so I can show up as my best self and be fully authentic. I'm worth it."

"The thing that is really hard and really amazing, is giving up on being perfect and beginning the work of becoming yourself."
~ Anna Quindlen

How To Have Your Happy and Lose Weight Too

But how can you possibly practice feeling happy in your body when you haven't lost the weight yet and you're still trapped in a body that isn't perfect, thinner, better?

Some folks feel like appreciating their body is a "nice to have," but kinda fluffy.

"Sure there are ways I can appreciate my body now, but what I really actually want to lose weight. I want my clothes to fit, so all this talk about body appreciation is nice, but it's not going to help me lose weight."

How can you appreciate your body and want to change it at the same time? It can feel like the two thoughts are juxtaposed to each other.

Either...I can love my body and be happy with how it is (which I am not)....or....I can want to lose weight and feel motivated to change.

I'd like to suggest that there is a way to hold both ideas in your head at the same time and they can both be true at the same time. It's possible because of "states and stages."

A state is how you feel at any moment (happy, sad, nervous, etc.). A stage is a measure of growth or progress (development over time).

For example:

Let's say you're sitting there, reading this book, and I said, "I want you to think of something that makes you feel happy." You might be able to think of a person or a circumstance that makes you happy or recall a happy memory. You might smile or feel a warm glow as you think about those things.

Or let's say I asked you to imagine something that makes you feel scared. You might be able to imagine standing on the edge of a cliff with no railing. Go ahead and imagine that now. Often, you'll feel a tingle in your palms as they start to sweat. You were able to have a physical reaction to a thought and feeling in your mind, while nothing changed in your external world.

So your "state" is an internal feeling and is something you can change based on what you choose to focus your thoughts on. It can change from moment to moment, no matter where you are or what you're doing.

Next let's look at stages.

Still sitting there, reading this book, imagine I asked you to become a world class tennis player. Is that something you can do or become in this moment?

Not so much.

You'd need to progress through the stages of beginner tennis player, intermediate, advanced, etc. You'd need to grow into a world class tennis player over time.

So how does this apply to weight loss?

You can choose to cultivate the emotional and mental state of love and appreciation for your body at the same time as wanting to progress to a different stage of weight loss.

You can want to change your body, AND marvel at the miracle it is at the same time. In fact, I'd say that the ONLY way to create sustainable, lifelong change is to proactively spend time feeling good about your body as you're losing weight.

One of my clients articulated it beautifully when he said this:

"There is no light at the end of the tunnel. You are responsible for
the light. I expected a treasure chest of gold and a crowd cheering
kind of moment when I lost the weight. It's not that at all.
It's easing into a place where you ask yourself,
Why don't I just choose to be happy?"
~Dr. Bob Thompson

If you never practice feeling good about your body, you can lose the weight, but you still find the flaws because that is all you've trained your brain to look for. If you want to make lasting change that sticks, you've got to practice feeling the way you want to feel now as you're practicing the tangible skills that allow your body to be at its ideal weight. The two go hand in hand.

Your mind and your body are the only things that will always be with you. Not your house, your job, or your clothes.

Taking time to invest in your relationship with yourself and your body is the best return in investment you can ever make.

Stairway To Heaven

Just like practicing a sport or learning to play an instrument, appreciating yourself is a practice, not a one-time item to check off on your to do list or something with a finish line.

Have you ever received a compliment and found it hard to believe it or let it sink in? Your partner can tell you all day long how gorgeous you are. But if you don't believe it in your mind, then it won't matter. You have to change your thought process. It doesn't matter if you change your body if you don't change your mind.

We get to choose where we focus our attention. There will always be things about your body to focus on that are not perfect. And there will always be things about your body that are miraculous.

Those two can both be true at the same time. You get to choose which one you focus on.

If you're looking for reasons why weight loss is hard, or ways in which your body is imperfect, that's what your brain will find.

If you're looking for reasons why your body is a miraculous organism that is the vehicle through which you get to experience this amazing life, then that is what your brain will find.

Decide what you want to look for because you'll find it.

Confidence is not magic. It's learned.

By shifting the way you think, you can shift everything.

It's okay if you have to remind yourself constantly to be patient with the process. Embrace that.

In fact, remind yourself on purpose. Write a sticky note. Put a reminder in your phone.

Remember, the primitive part of your brain is always scanning for what's wrong. That means that, left to its own devices, your brain will default toward the negative. So if you're gonna think a positive, helpful thought, you've gotta do so ON PURPOSE.

Just like you'd do reps with weights to get your muscles stronger, you can do reps with your brain to make positive thoughts stronger.

You may be thinking "Okay, that kinda makes sense...but this sounds a little too much like that airy fairy affirmation stuff."

Believe me, I've tried affirmations and discarded them because you can't put whipped cream on a pile of poop and call it ice cream.

Sometimes when you're having negative thoughts about yourself, it can be tough to just turn it around and think the opposite. Your brain won't believe it. Looking in the mirror and telling yourself that you're beautiful when you don't believe it feels frustrating and pointless.

Instead, focus on tiny baby step thoughts, or "stair step thoughts."

Imagine thoughts are on a set of stairs from negative at the bottom to positive at the top. Instead of trying to jump from the bottom step to the top step, you can move up gradually by taking the stairs one step at a time.

For example, if your thought is "I hate my body" you can't just tell yourself "I love my body" because your internal BS meter will know you don't believe it.

Instead, you can try a more neutral thought like "I have a body" because that feels "less bad" than the negative thought. And it feels true.

For example, you can take the thought "I hate my thighs" and turn it neutral by choosing the thought "I have thighs." Or from "None of my clothes fit!" to "I have clothes that I put on my body."

The key is that the neutral thought feels true. So it raises the vibration of how you're feeling about yourself without triggering your BS meter.

Here are two other strategies to try:

1) Use the word "but...."

   The word "but..." basically negates everything that was said before it.

   Imagine how not so great it would feel for your partner to say "I love you, but....." Whatever they say next negates the sentiment of "I love you."

   You can use that in the opposite direction too when you'd like to negate something less pleasant.

   Ex: *"I don't like the way I look in that picture, but I have made a lot of progress already."*

   or

   "I wish I hadn't eaten that cookie, but I am learning my triggers and making progress (no matter how small) all the time."

2) "I'm open to the idea that...."

   If you have an affirmation that you'd like to believe about yourself, but don't yet, you can use the phrase "I am open to the idea that....."

   For example, if you want to see yourself as strong and confident, but you don't see yourself that way now, you can try saying *"I am open to the idea that one day I can grow into the version of me that feels strong and confident."*

Stair step thoughts help you focus on where you're going, rather than where you are or where you've been.

Seems impossible? Let's explore....

Your body is a miracle in so many ways.

Without your body you would not be able to....

- see the glory of a sunset
- hug a loved one
- hear the laughter of a child
- feel the warmth of the sun on your shoulders
- smell the sweetness of the grass after the rain

....all our senses are a gateway to experience the beauty of this world. And you get to experience that because of your body.

Your body is intelligent.

For example:

- There are more neurons in the gut than in the brain. That's where the saying "a gut feeling" comes from.
- If you have children, your body knew how to create an entirely new human from just two cells coming together.
- Your body can heal itself when there's a cut or injury without any instruction from you.
- Your body keeps you alive while you sleep, protects you from infection, and warns you of danger.

Try completing this sentence:

I appreciate [X] about my body because of [ABC].

- I appreciate my hair because it has always been shiny and long and I like that about my hair.
- I appreciate my feet because even though they hurt sometimes, they get me where I want to go, and they give me freedom to experience this world that I would not have without my feet.

- I appreciate my arms because they allow me to hug my family and feel the softness of my dog's fur and those are some things that I love in this experience of life.

What are the things you love? Coffee? Going to the beach? Music?

How can you tap into all your senses? Not just what you see in the mirror. Think of the smell of coffee and that warmth of the mug in your hands. Imagine the feel of the sand between your toes or the cool water. Feel the beat of the music and how it moves you. Your body and all your senses are what bring those amazing things to you.

You and your body are going to be together for a long time.

What if you could create a partnership with your body that allows you to work together instead of fighting against each other?

How can you look in the mirror this week and look for what is right about you?

We only get to be in our bodies for a limited time.
Why not celebrate the journey instead of just riding it out
until it's over?
~Jen Sincero

TAKE IT FURTHER

Go to https://confidentbody.coach/book/ to download a body appreciation meditation, along with other bonuses.

Here are some ideas for how to make a measurable goal around practicing gratitude or body appreciation.

- Each day choose one body part and find something you appreciate about it (Ex: "I appreciate my eyes because they allow me to see my partner's smile.")
- Think of one thing you got to do today because of your body ("I heard my kids laughing today. I appreciate that my body allows me to hear that beautiful sound.")
- Whenever you eat, take a minute to notice that your body automatically sifts through the nutrients in that food and keeps the good stuff and gets rid of the rest.
- If you're hot and your body sweats, even if you hate sweating, that's an opportunity to feel grateful for your body's internal temperature regulation system that keeps you alive.

"I finally realized that being grateful to my body was key to giving more love to myself."
~Oprah Winfrey

CHAPTER 4
HOW TO MAKE FAILURE YOUR FRIEND

The Imperfect Race

By 2008, Heather Dorniden was already a decorated athlete. In her early years, she had been the Minnesota high school track and field state champion in both the 400m and 800m races. She had set school and state records in the process. When she was a freshman at the University of Minnesota, she was the NCAA Indoor Track and Field Champion in the 800 meter race.

So by the time she lined up to run the 600m race of the 2008 the Big Ten finals, there were high expectations that she'd finish first.

As the gun went off, she started off strong. She quickly passed the runner from the University of Indiana. The runner from Penn State was running a strong race out in front. After the first lap, Heather was in second place, behind the runner from Penn State.

Just as she neared the end of the second lap, she made her move. She pulled even with the runner from Penn State and pulled into first place. With only one lap to go, all she had to do was hold on to her lead.

But then, the worst happened.

Just as she passed the lead runner, Heather's front foot caught on her back foot, and she fell. Hard.

Heather knew from her training to get back up quickly. But once she was back on her feet, the other runners were already 30 meters ahead of her. All that ground she had fought so hard to win, was lost in a moment.

"After I fell, it was as if a vacuum had sucked all the energy out of the place."[7] Heather recalled.

It would have been easy for Heather to quit. These were the best runners across the conference. They would be tough to beat, without a 30-meter head start and only one lap to go. She had all the reason in the world to think, *"I guess this isn't my day."*

But she didn't.

She got up and kept going.

With only ½ a lap to go, she was still in last place, but gaining ground. With ⅓ of a lap to go, she passed one runner.

As she rounded the curve of the final home stretch, she was in third place with two runners still ahead of her.

Ten meters from the finish line, she passed the runner from Indiana University to take second place.

By any measure, her race was a gutsy effort and certainly a success.

And she kept going.

---

7   https://btn.com/2015/06/03/a-race-to-remember-i-had-no-idea-i-fell-like-that-in-inspirational-2008-run/

With three strides to go, she caught up to the lead runner. At two strides, they were dead even. With the final stride of the race, Heather pulled ahead of the final runner and finished in first!

She. Just. Kept. Going.

If Heather had let the mistake define her race, she could have quit. She could have stopped trying. Instead, she chose to keep going, despite the mistake.

Before long, Heather's resilient effort inspired others from all sorts of different backgrounds, who reached out to her to share their stories.

"This race is so easily relatable to everyone's lives. I've heard from cancer survivors, people battling addiction, struggling artists, parents, athletes and coaches of every sport, runners of every age and ability... the list could go on. I always tell people this race isn't just about never giving up, it's about discovering what you're capable of when you are given the opportunity to rise above adversity[8]." ~Heather Dorinden Kampf

Winning in weight loss is not a matter of running the perfect race with no mistakes. Every weight loss success has mistakes in it. Ev-er-y single one. Winning is a matter of persevering through the mistakes.

When we go on a diet, we tend to think that we have to follow it perfectly or we've failed. It's either perfect or it's a failure. There's no in between. We go a couple of days of being on track. Then we miss a day. We vow to start fresh the next day. But by 4:37 p.m. that resolve begins to crumble.

---

8   https://www.godupdates.com/christian-athlete-heather-dorniden-falls-wins/

We create meaning around our mistakes. When we make mistakes, we feel that we've failed and that we're hopeless. Eventually this leads to a constant cycle of starting - failing - stopping - starting all over from scratch. So much of our journey becomes about the rebooting and that's incredibly unproductive.

You don't need to reset and start all over again on New Year's Day, or Monday, or any other day.

In fact, mistakes are not "just part of the process that you need to get through." Instead, mistakes are a crucial part of the learning process of weight loss. You cannot succeed long term without the missteps and the learning.

Mistakes aren't failures! Mistakes are opportunities. They are the all-important stepping stones that guide you from where you are to where you want to be.

Making mistakes is how you learn to look at what happened with curiosity rather than judgment, learn about yourself and your triggers, and gather data to help you the next time you face something similar in the future.

The only true mistake is when you use a misstep as evidence for why you can't succeed. You cannot talk to yourself that way. The dialog in your head is crucial.

The Meta Skill

If there is ONE KEY SKILL of weight loss that can change everything for you, it is this:

Learn to look at each mistake, slip up, overeat, extra slice of birthday cake, etc. and ask yourself with compassionate curiosity, "What can I learn from that?"

It can feel demoralizing to think, "Oh I've been here before. Lose a little weight and then life happens, or we go on a trip and it all crumbles." That can be totally frustrating!

But you don't have to look at it that way. Instead, you can see every mistake as a gift. You get to turn it into an opportunity.

When I was in high school, my mom said that school was less about WHAT I was learning and more about "LEARNING HOW TO LEARN." She helped me realize that learning the system or the pathway to improvement is just as important as learning the subject matter itself.

That's what you're doing here.

The pathway of weight loss is:

1) Try something new
2) Mess up
3) Ask yourself with kindness, curiosity, and compassion, "What can I learn from this?"
4) Use that answer to inform future choices
5) Repeat

THAT is the meta skill of weight loss. If you can keep doing that one thing CONSISTENTLY, all the other things will fall into place over time.

You're not going to make great choices at every moment. That's normal. When that happens (because you can expect it to happen) go back and ask, "I wonder why I made that choice. I wonder what happened. What was the other choice I wish I had made? What could I have been thinking and feeling to make the better choice at that moment?"

IMPORTANT NOTE: No shame self-talk allowed.

Remember the Shame Spiral of Doom? That's not what we're doing here.

It's no wonder we feel lousy when we tell ourselves, "I always fail" or, "I always make the wrong choice." How is replaying that failure in your head helpful? You can't tell yourself, "I always fail" and expect to magically succeed. It doesn't work that way. Learn from the past, but don't live there.

TAKE IT FURTHER

For further examples on how to make failure your friend, go to https://confidentbody.coach/book/.

Life has ups and downs and sometimes our eating does too. Over time, when those ups and downs of life come at you, gradually you can begin to have a better conversation with yourself.

Those ups and downs are an important part of the process. They are not something to get upset about. They are an invitation to examine what's going on and come up with ideas and solutions to try out.

Failure is simply an education in what not to do. It's about discovery.

When things happen in your life, don't ask, "Why is this happening to me?" Instead ask "How is this happening for me?"

"Anyone who's never made a mistake has never tried anything new."
~Albert Einstein

The Learning Spiral

I don't know about you, but I get frustrated when I find myself needing to re-learn something I've already learned in the past. For example, travel is great, but I find it to be a little stressful. My brain defaults to wanting a glass of wine (or two) to settle down from the stress of travel.

I know this.

And yet, I still find myself having to re-learn the same lesson every time I travel.

I used to beat myself up over that. I mean how hard is it to learn something and remember it? It's like 2 steps forward and 1 step back. However, I decided that a better way to look at it is like a learning spiral.

I imagine walking a spiral staircase and on the first floor is lesson 101. As I travel along, it's normal to forget some of the things I've learned in the past. But as I keep walking, I get to the same topic at a new level. I'm re-learning some of the things I've learned before and adding new understanding on top of old knowledge when I reach lesson 201. And so on.

So if you're like me and find yourself needing to learn the same thing over and over again, don't fret. Instead of berating yourself for not learning your lesson, choose to see yourself getting a master's degree in the lessons on life. Getting smarter and wiser all the time, even if you need to re-learn some things along the way.

Thinking On Purpose

Sure, it's great to look at what feels like failure and say, "It's an opportunity!" But that doesn't mean the feelings like regret, guilt, and shame that come along with our perceived failure just magically go away.

What do you do with those feelings?

If you want better feelings, think better thoughts.

Your brain is the most powerful tool you have. If you don't manage it, it will manage you.

I once heard the analogy that our thought patterns are like ski tracks in the snow of our brains. Tracks that are well worn are really grooved in there. When you're on that track, the walls of the track are higher and harder to get out of.

Your brain doesn't care about your fulfillment, finding your passion, or looking smokin' hot in a bikini. It doesn't care about you creating a contribution to the world.

Your brain only cares about keeping you alive and doing so as efficiently as possible. So it's always looking for the old track.

When you're trying to create a new pattern, that's like a new track in the snow. There's not much of a groove yet, so it's easy to veer off course. You've got to practice it to make it stick.

We already know how the brain's natural default pattern will look for what's negative. Those old negative default thought patterns are like music playing in the background of your mind.

However, just because you're not paying attention to your thoughts doesn't mean there's no music playing. Without tuning the channel to what you WANT to listen to, it's like the radio dial in your brain is forever stuck on Rick Astley singing "Never Gonna Give You Up." (Great, now that's in my head. Ugh.)

You get to choose what thoughts get programmed on repeat. You can let the default muzak of your brain run wild, or you can proactively change the station to thoughts you WANT to listen to.

When was the last time you heard someone say, "You know, it's funny. Without really trying to change my thinking at all, I just found myself just feeling awesome and taking action on the things that matter most to me in life."

Ninety-five percent of your actions (and thus 95% of your results) are dictated by beliefs that are beneath your awareness in the subconscious mind. Do you really want to leave all that up to chance?

This is why it is super important to use that 5% of proactive thought to practice the thoughts you WANT to have and thereby influence what's under the surface.

Imagine if Oprah had listened to her default thoughts and never purposefully programmed her mind with empowering thoughts of making a difference in the world? Imagine what you could do if you took charge of your default thoughts and pur- pose- fully programmed them toward world altering greatness. (I'll show you how to do that in Chapter 8 with your redirect routine for self-sabotaging thoughts.)

If you were trying to learn how to shoot a basketball, how many times would you expect to need to practice before you start- ed to get proficient at it?

—> Habits of thought are the same way. We can't just hope our way to better thinking. We need to practice it, proactively.

Hoping your thoughts will improve on their own is like hoping you'll get better at shooting a basketball while sitting on the couch watching The Walking Dead.

You're not weak for needing to remind your brain of something you want to think on purpose. We tell our kids things over and over again. We don't question the need for repetition when we're trying to teach a child something new. (Potty training comes to mind.)

And yet we don't give ourselves the same grace. I can listen to one podcast and think, "I'm good. I've got it. I'm an adult. I've internalized it. I only need to do that once and I'll change my life."

But it doesn't work that way. It takes repetition. It takes intention. It's the sticky notes on the wall. The paper clip chain. The sticker on a chart. We jump from thing to thing to thing. But we don't repeat one thing enough.

Thanks to neuroplasticity, you can physically change your brain by changing your thoughts.

At the same time, we're literally rewiring neural pathways here, people! It takes time. You have to do it over and over and over.

Sherlock Holmes Your Way to Success

I always liked math….until it came time to take calculus.

Math used to come easy to me, and suddenly I was having to work really hard just to pass the class.

I was one of the lucky ones. I had fifth period math with Mrs. Onorati instead of second period with Mr. Smith.

Mrs. Onorati was one of those wonderful teachers that cared more about her students loving learning than about catching you in a mistake. She made us show our work because she was always looking for ways to give partial credit. She was looking for evidence that we had at least some understanding of the math concepts, even if we didn't get the numerical answer exactly right.

When we operate with a perfection mindset, then there's no room for partial credit. That's like saying, "If I can't get 100% on my calculus test, then I'm not even going to answer the rest of the questions."

What?!? That's crazy talk!

Why can't we be that favorite teacher to ourselves?

The way to rewire those neural pathways in your brain is not to look for perfection. It is to look for evidence of little ways that you're making progress.

What if showing your work counts?

What if effort counts?

Grade yourself on a curve.

Give yourself points for showing up and doing the work, even if you didn't do it perfectly.

Even if the scale didn't move. (Especially if the scale didn't move!)

Purposefully look for ways to make your success feel as amazing to yourself as you can. It's not enough to simply want to feel good about the progress you've made. It takes conscious effort to look for what's right and to celebrate the small actions you're taking to change your life.

You've got to LOOK FOR EVIDENCE.

Be like Sherlock Holmes finding those little clues that point to your eventual success. Look for clues and confirmations that you're on the right track. Proof won't just show up at your door. You've got to go out and look for it.

What is the best form of evidence? Effort.

You can always find little ways that you are making an effort to be kind to yourself. Highlight those in your mind as much as you can.

With the old diet mentality, you might think, "I walked two miles and ate salad for lunch today. I followed my plan. And I've only lost one pound. What am I doing wrong? This is why I hate the scale. I think my body just isn't able to lose weight."

With that kind of thinking, success is staring you in the face, and yet all you see is how it's not working.

Remember: Whatever you're looking for, you'll find it.

Even a radiologist, who's very profession is to look and find things, can miss something obvious if they're looking for something else. A study done by Trafton Drew, an attention researcher at Harvard Medical School, found that when radiologists were looking for cancer nodules in scans of lungs, 83% of them missed an image of a gorilla embedded in the scan.[9]

When you have told your brain to look for one thing, you miss the other things that are right in front of you. When you're

---

9   Why even radiologists can miss a gorilla hiding in plain sight.

looking for what's wrong with you, you miss all the things that are right with you.

Moments like that are an opportunity to be proud of showing up for yourself today. Instead of wasting your precious energy thinking about all of the ways that progress doesn't matter, you get to decide how you want to think about your weight loss each week. You need to celebrate yourself all the time for the little things you ARE doing to make progress.

Instead of thinking, "I only lost one pound this week" you could tell yourself, "I changed my life this week. I'm drinking water. I'm making meal plans. I'm walking every day."

I'm serious. Those little wins are so important.

Because those little wins give your brain a hit of dopamine, the feel good chemical. The helps you brain remember "Hey, I like this." And then that fuels your motivation to keep going.

If you skip right past small wins and don't take time to celebrate or congratulate yourself, then the brain doesn't get that dopamine. It doesn't remember why it wants to keep working so hard, and thus motivation wanes.

Feeling good is the fuel that runs the engine of motivation. Give yourself the best chance to feel good and keep firing that engine of motivation by getting excited about the things that ARE within your control.

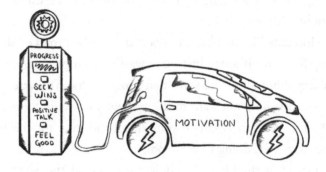

Fueling the Engine of Motivation

Take credit and ownership for all you've accomplished without giving yourself a hard time for not having accomplished it sooner or made different choices in the moment.

Own how far you've come given where you ARE rather than where you want to get to.

You cannot hate on the work you've already done or the number of pounds you've already lost (as if they are not enough). You have got to make your progress sound as impressive to yourself as you can.

Why is this so important?

In her book *The Progress Principle*[10] Teresa Amabile explains that human beings are actually more motivated by progress toward the goal than by the achieving goal itself. If you want to make it easier to keep going, you've got to allow yourself to feel like you're making progress.

Talking up your successes to yourself makes you feel like a badass, and you can go out and do anything. Downplaying your

---

10 The Progress Principle by Teresa Amabile

progress makes you feel like you're not doing enough. Which one do you think is going to make you want to keep going?

TAKE IT FURTHER

For ideas and examples on how to look at your actions this week and highlight them to yourself in the most positive way possible, check out https://confidentbody.coach/book/.

The reason why this is so important is so that you don't give up.

If you give up, you guarantee that you won't succeed. And if you're hard on yourself in those tough moments, then you'll have less motivation to keep going.

However, if you can give yourself hope in those moments that you're still making imperfect progress, then you'll feel more motivated to keep going.

When you give yourself the gift (and I'm serious, it's truly a gift) of allowing yourself to look for ways that you're proud of your progress, no matter how small, you are putting gas in the engine that keeps you going.

That feeling of, "Hey, I'm doing a good job!" is what helps you keep going when you don't have your favorite day, or you are wondering, "Is this even worth it?"

Those little wins that you're proactively looking for are proving to your subconscious one little win at a time that you CAN do this, you CAN make progress, and you can blow your mind of what you're capable of.

The more you proactively, purposefully program your brain and look for ways that you do make good choices, the more it will begin to filter for those examples.

The more evidence you begin to accumulate, the more belief you begin to develop that maybe you actually CAN do positive actions that eventually result in losing weight.

Weight loss is a RESULT. Results happen after a series of positive actions.

You can't ignore the actions and hope for a positive result.

First focus on the actions and then the results will begin to take care of themselves.

It's like lifting weights in the gym...

If you want a strong body, you gotta lift heavy things intentionally.

If you want better thoughts, you gotta look for them and think them intentionally!

Hope is a discipline.

Any positive thought or feeling is a discipline.

You've got to be your own biggest cheerleader!

Your success depends on it.

I Need a Hero

When my kids were little, they would ask to listen to the Kids' XM radio station on the way to kindergarten. Fortunately, kids' music has come a long way since "The Wheels on the Bus Go Round And Round."

One of my favorite songs was "The Princess Who Saved Herself" by Jonathan Coulton[11]. In it, the princess lives on her own so she does whatever she wants to. She eats cake, plays guitar, and never wears socks.

When a dragon comes around, she catches it by the tail, and they end up having tea. When the pretentious prince calls, she doesn't have time for him. She gives the Evil Witch a makeover and they all end up starring in a band called The Kingdom of the Princess Who Saved Herself.

The princess tells herself a different story. She doesn't need a handsome prince to come save her. Because she saves herself. How about you? What story are you telling yourself?

You don't have to be a novelist or a songwriter to be pretty good at telling stories. In fact, we all tell ourselves stories in our mind to explain our lives.

You are the main character in the story of your life. But what role are you playing? Are you a victim or the hero?

When you look at what's happened in your life, in your childhood, or what you ate last weekend, ask yourself "So what? What am I making that mean?"

You get to tell the story. You get to make up the meaning you give to everything. You can make it mean something terrible or something amazing.

You can make last weekend's slip-up mean that you're a failure and you'll never lose weight. Or you can make it mean that

---

11 https://www.jonathancoulton.com/2010/08/16/the-princess-who-saved-herself/

you learned something. You're wiser for it and more prepared for next time.

What is the story that empowers you?

How can you be the hero of your own story?

The only difference is what you decide to focus on. So no matter what's going on in your life, no matter how many times you've tried to lose weight and think you "failed," and no matter what you ate last weekend, I encourage you to ask yourself "So what? What am I making it mean and what do I WANT to make it mean?"

Maybe every time you tried to lose weight in the past was simply a practice run helping you learn what doesn't work for you, just like Thomas Edison learning lots of ways how not to make a light bulb.

Instead of wallowing in guilt and self-recrimination, imagine this as just an early chapter in your story.

The story where you overcame challenges and setbacks and little by little began to make progress, changing tiny habits here and there. In this story, you learned to adjust the way you think about things gradually. Over time you lost [X] number of pounds and now you keep it off year after year because you learned to change your thinking and your behavior, rather than simply following "the rules" of yet another diet.

This is your story.

Can you see yourself telling someone that story someday? The story of how you lost your weight and how you maintain it for good?

Don't hold out for a hero. Be one for yourself.

CHAPTER 5
HOW TO CHANGE YOUR HABITS

Why Diets Go Against the Grain

When I was eleven years old, my family packed up the old 1983 Ford station wagon (affectionately known as the Dragon Wagon) and headed down to Hawks Cay in Key Largo, FL.

We had our swimsuits, diving fins, the fishing poles, towels, sunscreen, the works. Once Dad hitched up the 18-ft Aquasport outboard motorboat behind the car, we were ready to go!

We were approximately seven minutes into the four-hour drive when a car slammed on their brakes in front of us as we approached a light.

Dad hit the brakes HARD. But the extra weight of the boat behind us kept us right on going.

The tires screeched.

Smoke billowed out from beneath the car as we came to a stop barely inches from the bumper in front of us.

Whew! That was close.

Your brain can be a lot like my dad driving our station wagon with a heavy boat behind it.

There is a common analogy that describes the relationship between the conscious and subconscious mind like an elephant and its rider. The rider has the brains, but the elephant has the brawn. Or in our case, Dad was the rider, and the boat was the elephant.

How many times have you started out strong on a diet, only to lose steam around week three or four? The novelty wears off. Your willpower begins to drain, and before long, you're back to your old ways.

What is the secret to maintaining momentum past weeks three to four?

It all comes down to your subconscious mind.

The subconscious mind is much more powerful than the conscious mind, just like the elephant is more powerful than the rider. We make the decision to "lose weight" or "go on a diet" with our conscious mind. But the everyday actions are most often dictated by the subconscious mind.

The subconscious evolved at a time when any change in the environment could mean danger. Since a diet is all about changing your behaviors, your subconscious mind sees a diet as a threat.

Keeping things the same is safe. Our biology actively seeks to keep us at "normal," which means our old weight and our old patterns. So a diet goes against the grain of how we are wired.

How do we make changes in our actions and habits that don't get derailed by the subconscious mind?

The key is to make change small enough so that it doesn't trigger the subconscious mind to freak out.

1) Small changes fly under the radar of your subconscious mind's change-o-meter and thus they don't set off the self-sabotaging alarm bells.

2) Small changes are easier to sustain and help you change the way you see yourself over time.

3) Small changes don't feel like deprivation. The destination always feels like the journey did. If you're making yourself miserable on the way down the scale, you're going to be miserable trying to stay there. Small changes don't feel miserable. They feel doable.

Fad diets promise results quickly.

But it is REALLY hard to sustain those fad diets because they ask you to change too many things all at once and that works directly against the way your brain is wired to accept (or not accept) change.

You can willpower your way to big changes for a short time and that can lead to fast results. However, the subconscious mind will always be working to get things "back to the way they were" because that is what the mind sees as "safe."

Diets fail because they don't address the underlying mental scripts and subconscious behaviors.

Want my advice?

Never try to fix everything all at once. Being overwhelmed does not help you achieve your goals.

Simplicity does.

1% - Tiny or Infinite?

The problem is small changes aren't exciting. We don't see progress right away, so we give up.

Most of the time, the way we think about change is that we're not close to the goal until we're close to the goal. For example, if I want to lose fifty pounds, I'm close to my goal once I've lost forty-five pounds, not three pounds.

We think that the first few steps don't count. We don't give ourselves credit for creating a meal plan and following it 20% of the time because that's not close to perfect.

We need to look at change differently.

The biggest leap is from zero to one. The difference between doing something and nothing is everything. From zero to one is the part that most people never do. The difference between nothing and a little bit is infinite.

From zero to one is the hard part. Once you've gotten going, it's just rinse and repeat from there. The hardest part of a run is getting out the door. The hardest part of meal planning is sitting down to do it.

Perfectionism keeps us thinking that doing a little is pointless. We are too busy, too tired, too stressed to try imperfectly. But doing the tiniest step imperfectly consistently adds up much faster than doing perfect steps once or twice, and then quitting.

Doing a little is EVERYTHING. If you spend 1% of your time or effort making yourself a little better, over a year you'll be exponentially closer to your goal. It's just math. 1% compounded over 365 days creates exponential progress.

- $1.01^{365} = 37.78$
- $1.00^{365} = 1$
- $0.99^{365} = 0.03$

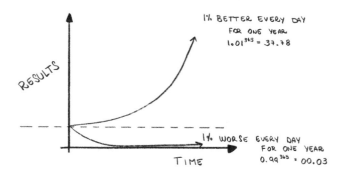

1% TINY OR INFINITE?

RESULTS

1% BETTER EVERY DAY
FOR ONE YEAR.
$1.01^{365} = 37.78$

1% WORSE EVERY DAY
FOR ONE YEAR
$0.99^{365} = 00.03$

TIME

While doing something small seems insignificant, the space between the person doing nothing and the person doing something is huge. Give yourself the chance to just be 1% better consistently, and you'll be amazed how much change you can make over time.

Change your definition of success. If you define success as progress, then even if you stumble forward, you're still further ahead than you were before.

Making progress your goal changes the internal story from "not good enough" to "better than yesterday."

How To Simplify Habit Change

1) Make It Easier to Start

In 1947, the world was rebuilding after WWII. The United States had a vested interest in Japan's economic recovery, so the US government sent visionary business and academic figures to Japan to help get their economy back on track.

He didn't know it at the time, but one man would have a massive impact on the economies of both Japan and the US with just one small idea.

W. Edwards Deming[12] introduced the idea of testing small changes to deliver improvement on manufacturing processes. The Japanese saw how increasing quality with small changes led to decreased expenses over time. They embraced the process and refined it, calling it "kaizen" for "continuous improvement."[13]

In 1950, the Toyota Corporation embraced kaizen fully and began their quest toward dominating the world of automobile manufacturing. Based on the number of Camrys and Priuses out there, it pretty much worked.

In a nutshell kaizen means: Small changes done CONSISTENTLY over time accumulate and lead to huge shifts.

What works in business works in weight loss too.

Kaizen is the antidote to the diet mentality.

- Diets ask you to make big changes, but small things will get in the way.

---

12 https://www.creativesafetysupply.com/articles/a-brief-history-of-kaizen-the-key-players/
13 https://crm.org/articles/the-history-of-kaizen

- Kaizen asks you to make small changes, and big things result.

Why do small changes succeed where big changes fall off the wagon?

The amygdala is the part of the brain where the fight or flight response lives. Because a diet changes so many things, it triggers the amygdala to set off warning bells to either fight or run from the changes you're trying to make. No wonder we fall off the (station) wagon!

Kaizen is stealthy. It's like sneaking back in the house after curfew and getting past your dad sleeping on the couch without waking him up. Small changes get around the amygdala because small, easily achievable steps help you tiptoe past the fight or flight response.

Over time, as the small steps continue, your brain gets used to them. Repetition creates new neural wiring and builds new habits. Gradually, the brain's resistance to change weakens.

Activation Energy

A long time ago, I used to teach middle school science. We covered everything from earthquakes and volcanoes to the basics of chemistry. My favorite part was mixing vinegar and baking soda and watching the bubbles fizz up out of a paper mache volcano.

During my time teaching, I learned something interesting about chemical reactions. When two reactants come together (like vinegar and baking soda) it takes energy in order to get them to bond and change into the products (the bubbles and fizz). That energy is called activation energy.

Imagine rolling a large rock up a hill. It takes a lot of work to get the rock up the hill! But once you get to the peak, it'll roll down and break apart on its own. Activation energy is the work it takes to get the rock up the hill.

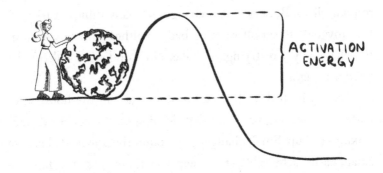

ACTIVATION ENERGY

Habits require activation energy too. The more complex or daunting the habit, the higher the hill you're trying to climb.

Let's say you create a goal for yourself to run three miles five days a week before the kids get up. That's like trying to roll a boulder the size of a car up Mt. Kilimanjaro.

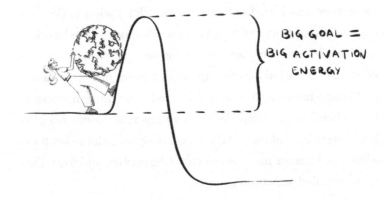

BIG GOAL = BIG ACTIVATION ENERGY

Why not make it easier on yourself by choosing a smaller rock to roll up a smaller hill?

Choose a smaller rock by making success tiny.

- Losing fifty pounds feels hard. Losing two pounds feels doable.
- Doing an intense 38-minute HIIT workout feels hard. Putting on my shoes and hitting play on the video feels easy.
- Planning my meals for the whole week feels hard. Planning my dinner tonight feels reasonable.
- Feeling all my feelings feels hard. Allowing my feelings for one minute feels attainable.

The idea is to create a habit. Habits are created with repetition. If you can repeat a small action, then you can build on it.

Some days the only change is eating a little less ice cream or walking to the mailbox. Make micro changes and do them consistently when the big changes are too daunting. Overcome activation energy by lowering the goal to something that you can do in two minutes.

- Do one stretch.
- Walk to the mailbox and back.
- Put on your exercise clothes.
- Ask yourself "What's the smallest thing I can do today feel good?"

Don't look for the seven-foot bar to jump over. Find the one-foot bar and step over it consistently.

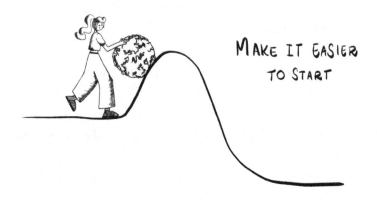

MAKE IT EASIER TO START

2) Make It Easier to Succeed

A perfectionist can do eighty sit ups and still feel like a failure because they didn't do 100. This hurts your long-term progress because it feels lousy to be falling short.

Choose a smaller hill by making success binary. It's like a light switch. The switch is either on or off. Meaning you either did a sit up or you didn't. There is no "grade" for a good workout versus a bad one.

- Did I get my running shoes on? Y/N?
- Did I meditate for at least one minute? Y/N?
- Did I plan any meals this week? Y/N?
- Did I eat any veggies today at all? Y/N?

The process is where the gold is. If you can win the process, the results will take care of themselves. When creating a new habit, the goal is to groove in the practice first, and then level up the challenge of it.

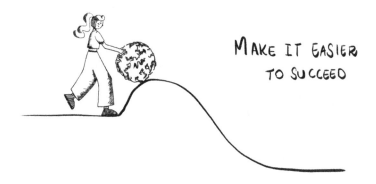

MAKE IT EASIER
TO SUCCEED

3) Make It Easier to Keep Going

What's more important to weight loss: Commitment or consistency?

Whenever a workout program asked me to decide, "How committed are you to this change?" on the outside I'd be like "I'm all in!…sorta" I mean, that's what you're supposed to say, right?

But on the inside, I'd be thinking "Honestly, I'm kinda scared that I can't keep this up. And I'm afraid to admit that to myself, much less say it out loud."

Have you ever felt that way?

Over time, I've become a much bigger fan of focusing on consistency rather than commitment.

If there's ever a goal or a change that you're not totally sure you're committed to, great! That is a sign to cut the goal in half.

Then cut it in half again.

Don't beat yourself up for not choosing a big, audacious goal. Instead, congratulate yourself for finding a boundary of where your current commitment limits are and stay just inside them.

Any change you consider ought to be one you can see yourself still doing consistently five years from now.

What if you worried less about weight loss and simply focused on micro changes that were easy enough that you knew you could keep doing them consistently?

The big changes are hard to keep up consistently. When you're inconsistent, that feels like failure. When you feel like a failure, you want to quit. So set up the system in a way that makes it easy to keep going.

Lower your expectations out of love for yourself! We usually set the bar high out of self-loathing. Set the bar lower to give yourself a chance to win. When you set the bar low enough, then self-doubt won't stop you.

By making success easier to achieve, you get to focus on progress and consistency, rather than perfect results. It allows you to take more action with less fear.

Little changes provide evidence to your brain that you can commit to a change. This process helps you to finally break the cycle of making promises to yourself that you don't keep. By keeping the changes small, you're making commitments to yourself that you can keep doing for the rest of your life.

"By the yard, it's hard. By the inch, it's a cinch!"
~Robert Mauer

Imagine an airplane is flying from Los Angeles to New York. The plane doesn't make one huge turn toward New York and then coast from there. In fact, for most of the trip, the plane is slightly off course.

Along the way, the pilot makes small shifts to course correct to get the plane closer and closer to the destination. There are no big changes, just CONSISTENT tiny little adjustments.

Health and weight loss can be the same way. By going on a diet, you're telling the brain, "We're changing the way we do things around here, people!" But that doesn't work. As soon as you slip up and eat some cheesecake, it's too easy to say, "Well, I blew it. I guess I'm off my diet."

When you focus on making small changes along the way, if you have the cheesecake, you can learn from it and make a course correction the next time you're faced with a similar choice.

You don't have to change everything in order to be healthy and lose weight.

You just need to make little tweaks and adjustments, one at a time, that you can do over and over again. That's how behavior change begins to take hold. It's not about forcing yourself into yet another diet plan that won't stick.

Remember the Progress Principle? Feeling like you're "winning" is the fuel that runs the engine of motivation.

Because it's so important to be able to feel good about yourself, sometimes it can be useful to create a goal on a spectrum.

For example:

- "On my best days I'll strive for X. But if life doesn't go perfectly, I'll still be proud of myself for doing Y, which I feel confident I can accomplish even on my toughest days."

How would you feel about creating a goal you're reaching for and one you'd be happy with on days that life doesn't quite go to plan?

The key to successful change is feeling like you're making progress. Give yourself the best chance to feel successful, even when you don't live up to perfect expectations.

"Strive for continuous improvement rather than perfection."
~Kim Collins

One of the best ways to make it easier to keep going is to reduce the number of decisions you have to make.

Decisions make it harder to get the rock up the hill. They don't make the hill higher or the rock bigger. But they drain your willpower, so they make you weaker.

Having more choices is not necessarily a good thing. Choices drain our energy.

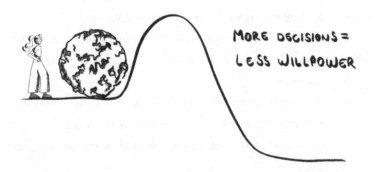

MORE DECISIONS = LESS WILLPOWER

Here's my inner monologue when I haven't planned ahead for a workout:

- Should I hit snooze or get up?
- What should I wear?
- Should I go to the gym or go for a run?
- Do I want to do cardio or lift weights?
- Or I could do an on-demand video at home.
- Or I could stay here in bed and keep thinking about it until I no longer have time to work out, and I might as well sleep until I need to get the kids up for school.

The harder I make my brain work, the more likely it is that I will hit the "Easy Button" and just lay in bed.

Enjoy the freedom of fewer choices.

Make a plan for what kind of exercise you want to do, when you need to start, and set out clothes so that all you need to do is get out the door.

It's the same with food. Pre-portion out serving sizes of veggies and put them in a ziplock bag. Then when you're hungry for a snack, all you need to do is grab the bag instead of having to take time to cut up vegetables.

Make it easier to just get going by doing less thinking.

Once you've rolled that rock up the hill, it's easier to keep it rolling in that direction. You just need to make it a lot easier to get the habit started by reducing the number of decisions.

4) Make It Easier to Feel Good

If you want healthy habits to not be a chore, you need to give your brain a reward for doing them. You can't expect to take away the natural reward that your brain used to get from the less-than-great habit, and have your brain be fine with it.

It's important to attach positive feelings to the action you're trying to groove in so that your brain will remember it likes this new habit. It's really hard to keep doing something you don't enjoy.

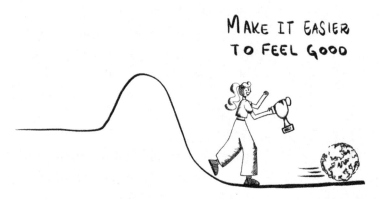

MAKE IT EASIER TO FEEL GOOD

Bad habits are easier to keep doing because they naturally give your brain a reward.

When you're trying to groove in a new habit, you need to proactively add in a reward so your brain will remember to want to do the new habit.

Your brain seeks pleasure and avoids pain. If there's a new thing you want to do, attach pleasure to it. Give yourself a win for accomplishing even the smallest of tasks.

Ex: After I ....[action you're trying to do], then I get to .... [small reward].

Ex: After I .... meditate for three minutes, then I ... get to have a cup of coffee.

How might you fill in the blanks above to attach the habit to something you already do and give yourself a small reward?

Here are some ideas:

- Keep a chart and give yourself a check or smiley face or a gold star sticker for every time you do the new habit.
- For every time you do the new habit, give yourself a non-food treat. Like five minutes of playing Candy Crush or a minute to look at kittens online
- Find a buddy or a friend to collaborate with you and create a collective goal where the two of you are working together to reach a bigger goal.
  - Ex: "Between the two of us, we're aiming to get up from our desks 20x this week." and have a spreadsheet to keep track and tally up the totals.

"Training your brain is like training a dog to sit or come or lie down. It's all about meaning, simplicity, treats, and repetition."
~Jen Sincero

As you're practicing habit change, it's important to make it easier to get started, easier to succeed, and easier to keep going.

And you need to make it easier to FEEL SUCCESSFUL.

Weight loss is not a straight line. It is a product of consistent behaviors. Get excited about the process, and less focused on the outcomes. Focus on feeling great about your progress, and the results will take care of themselves.

Habit Hacks

Talk to yourself with purpose

Some days, it's just plain hard to get going. It's too cold to work out. You're too tired to cook a healthy dinner. Sometimes healthy habits just are just plain hard.

In those moments, try NOT to stay present.

What?

That's right. Throw mindfulness and presence out the window.

Ignore the now and focus on the finish. "I'll feel so good after...." "I'll feel so proud of myself after...." "I can brag to my spouse after..." etc.

- Trying to get yourself to move more? Intentionally create the thought loop, "If I can just get started, I know I'll feel so awesome after my workout."
- Trying to drink more water? Remind yourself, "I'll feel better in my body after I drink this glass of water."
- Want to eat more veggies? Proactively tell yourself, "I'm crushing my goals like a boss, and I feel so virtuous and pious when I eat them."

What you focus on expands. Put your focus where your feel good is, or where it will be.

Harness existing momentum

I've started and stopped the habit of meditating like eight times. I'd get on a roll and then my schedule would be different one day and suddenly I'm out of the habit. I once came close to meditating every day for a year. Then the pandemic happened and even though I had more time than ever, I just couldn't seem to find the time to meditate.

When routines change, it's hard to keep habits going because the normal anchors we use to help trigger the habit are missing. That's why it's harder to meal plan on weekends and harder to exercise when you're on vacation. Your normal routine is disrupted, and thus the foundational supports of the habit are disrupted too.

Simply being aware of that can help you give yourself a little grace when life happens and the habit you're trying to establish gets pushed to the side. View it as a temporary disruption rather than an indictment on your ability to stick to something new.

Imperfect consistency is better than
a perfect habit abandoned.

In my opinion, consistency is less about doing something without fail every day. It's more about knowing that you give yourself grace to do it imperfectly as frequently as you can. If you miss a day, that's all right. Just try not to miss two in a row. Try not to let it mean anything.

Consistency is the antidote of perfection. It's about quantity, not quality. Imperfection is a beautiful thing!

Your current routines are like a big heavy train that has already gone through the process of getting moving, and now it's moving at full speed down miles of straightaway. The habit you're trying to create is like a heavy box car just sitting idle on the track. It takes a lot of energy to get it moving.

Harness the power of the train that is already running with at full speed by partnering the new habit with something you already do naturally.

It's really hard to get momentum going if each day you're asking yourself, "When am I going to meal plan today?" It's much easier if you can attach the new habit you're trying to create to something you already do.

For example, what is something you already do every day?

Drink coffee.

What habit are you trying to establish?

Plan my meals.

Introduce your existing habit to the new one you want to spend more time with.

- **After I .....[action you already do], then I will.....[action you want to do].**
  - ○ Ex: After I .... get up and use the restroom in the morning, then I will.... meditate for three min.
- **Before I .....[action you already do], then I will.....[action you want to do].**
  - ○ Ex: Before I ...brush my teeth at night, then I will... look for one thing I appreciate about my body.

**Remember to give your brain a little reward for completing the new habit!

Simple Doesn't Mean Easy

One of the things that drives me crazy about diet programs is they never tell you "Hey, just so you know, it's gonna get really hard around day six and you're going to want to eat your entire fridge by day nine (that is, if you make it that far)."

Keeping habit change simple is the key to success. However, simple and easy are not the same thing. Even though you're keeping things simple, obstacles will come up.

Your brain is extremely vested in keeping the status quo. Old habits are safe. Know up front that the subconscious mind is gonna put up some resistance to change.

That resistance sounds like....

1. The demanding, results-driven voice in your head.

   It takes patience and self-love and respect to tolerate that voice in your head that says, "We've been doing this for two days! Why isn't the scale moving? This isn't worth it." Thank you, Demanding Voice. Super helpful.

   We all have that voice. The one that is impatient and not okay with small changes. It's normal. Know that it'll be there, asking for daily proof that this is working.

   You know it's working because you're showing up every day. And on the days that you miss, you know it's no big deal because you can get back on track tomorrow. Know that you are strong enough to tolerate the negative voice that demands perfect results in less time.

2. Pessimism

   It can be hard to feel optimistic and confident that you're on the right track when the little steps you're taking are small, and it's tough to see measurable progress from day to day. It's tempting to protect yourself from potential failure. The brain is very good at throwing up warning signals that scream, "This isn't working!"

YOU ARE A MIRACLE

However, all that does is make you experience the feeling of failure in advance. Instead, if you choose to feel positive about the practice and celebrate the opportunity to make a choice for yourself, the outcome will take care of itself.

That's why it's so important to note the amazing things you are doing for yourself and count those as wins, rather than only looking toward the end result (which of course will come with time.)

3. Tolerating screw-ups

    Every single person who ever tried to change a habit did so imperfectly with lots of screw-ups along the way. However, it's really tempting to see those screw-ups as evidence for why you're not cut out for this and why you just don't have it in you.

    DO NOT LISTEN TO THAT VOICE! Change that channel!

    Screw-ups are like speed bumps through the parking lot on your way to the spa to get a massage. Yeah! Roll right over those suckers at 35 miles an hour. You can handle a bump when a massage is waiting for you.

All of those obstacles that your brain puts in the way of change are smoke screen what's quivering just beneath the surface.

Fear of failure.

Fear of failure is a totally normal human emotion. It's just your brain trying to protect you. It's doing its job! There's nothing wrong with you when your brain offers up thoughts that have some flavor of "What if I fail?"

Chances are you've learned from repeated experiences that attempting to lose weight means "failure". Failure feels really bad because of what we make it mean about ourselves.

It's no wonder that your subconscious mind would be sending up warning signals saying, "Oh hold up. We're tried this before. Not only did it not work, but it felt really lousy. Let's avoid this."

You don't have to fight thoughts like that. Just because your brain sends up a thought, doesn't make it true.

It's something you can welcome because it is reminding you to purposefully think the thoughts you WANT.

Thoughts like:

- "Even though past tries didn't work out the way I wanted, those were just practice runs. They taught me what doesn't work. It's all part of my ultimate success story."

- Or…"It's impossible for me to fail. I know I'll have slip-ups, but I now see those as learning opportunities instead of mistakes or failure. If I just keep going, success is inevitable."

What if you viewed each thought of fear as an invitation to change the channel? Instead of being afraid that you won't succeed, be afraid of being in the exact same place one year from now. If I try and fail, I grow. If I don't try, I stagnate.

Imagine it this way:

Let's say you're helping your child to learn how to ride a bike.

However, in the past, she had a crash and fall from her bike that left her feeling pretty afraid to try again.

What would you tell your child and how would you coach her to be able to ride a bike with confidence?

Fear of failure is normal. But you don't have to let it stop you. Keep rocking it. Don't give up.

God doesn't expect perfection. Just growth. Maybe that can be enough for us too.

You are not who you were yesterday.

Nor are you yet who you will be tomorrow.

You are in the beautiful middle in the process of becoming.

Each day, each choice, you're becoming the person you know is inside you.

The one who whispers, "I'm ready to shine my light into the world."

She's already there inside you. I see her. You are already her.

You are simply learning to uncover your strength and revealing her to yourself and the world, one choice at a time.

"You are the light of the world....let your light shine before others"
Matthew 5:14-15

CHAPTER 6
HOW TO SERIOUSLY, LIKE FOR REAL, CHANGE YOUR HABITS

Perception Is Reality

When I was in seventh grade, I tried out for the soccer team. One day the coach said, "Who wants to try being goalie?" I thought, "Why not? I like getting dirty." Since I was the only one still willing to play the position after day two, I got the job.

If you've ever seen or played soccer, you know that the players wear shin guards, and you need tall socks to cover them. The first time I played goalie, I didn't have any soccer socks yet, so I used an old pair of knee-high tube socks with three big green stripes at the top. (No one ever accused me of being stylish.)

In my first game wearing my old-school socks, I happened to play well and stopped a few goals. I was so elated (and surprised, since I was kinda terrified of the ball at that time), I decided that those knee-high, green striped, tube socks were my "lucky socks."

If my mom had known then that would mean she'd be washing the same pair of socks weekly for the next six years, she probably would have put the kibosh on the illusion of "luckiness" I bestowed on those socks.

Over the course of my soccer career, I wore those socks with great success. When I put on those socks, they gave me a sense of confidence. If someone came near my goal when I had my lucky socks on, the ball was mine. I played bigger and more aggressively when I took on the identity I felt the socks gave me.

Were the socks actually lucky? Or did I play better when wearing them because I thought they were lucky?

Scientists have done experiments to measure the impact of expectation on results. For example in one experiment, Japanese scientists rubbed poison ivy on the arms of participants and waited to see how long their skin broke out with a rash.[14] (Who would volunteer for such an experiment?!)

Here's the crazy thing: while the participants' skin did break out in a rash, the plant was not actually poison ivy.

In another experiment, scientists told hotel maids that their everyday work burned about the same number of calories as a true workout.[15] (I can 100% believe that. Cleaning the house is hard work!) A control group was not told anything about the calorie burn of their work. In the test group, even though they did nothing different, after a few weeks, the maids that thought they were burning more calories lost weight and reduced their BMI.

---

14 The A.P.P.L.E. Principle by Chris Estes
15 Mindset Matters https://www.eurekalert.org/news-releases/780734

What we perceive is happening can actually affect our experience of what happens. This is called Expectancy Theory.[16] Our expectation causes certain neurons to fire. Those neurons release neurotransmitters and hormones that literally impact the physiology of our bodies.

In other words, your beliefs strongly influence your results because they impact both your effort and your physiology.

The way you perceive the world and yourself in it becomes the story you tell yourself about reality. Over time, that story becomes your identity.

The self-identity you carry around in your head is very powerful. It can be empowering (like "I'm good at math") or disempowering (like "I'm always late").

Are these stories true?

Not necessarily, but you make them true the more you tell yourself the same story.

Beliefs are just thoughts that we've repeated over and over. And thoughts are just sentences in your mind.

Sentences are only true if we believe them.

For example:

"I believe in Santa Claus."

or

"I'm not enough as I am."

They're both just sentences. Neither is more or less true than the other. We give power to them only when we choose to believe them.

---

16 Expectancy Theory https://www.sciencedirect.com/topics/social-sciences/expectancy-theory

How you label yourself internally makes a huge difference in your success long term. Your subconscious mind makes sense of the world through the lens of your identity. Therefore, it is very invested in protecting and maintaining your identity as is.

When there is something you already believe, your brain is like a dog sniffing for a bone looking for examples to prove it true.

There are millions of bits of information coming at you every second. There's no way you could hold all of them in your awareness at once. So the brain has designed a filtering system called the Reticular Activating System (RAS) to filter out things that don't matter to you and highlight the ones that do.

If you tell yourself, "I'm always late" the RAS will highlight times when you were late and filter out times that you were actually on time.

A lot of times, the stories we tell ourselves come from past experience or from narratives we learned when we were growing up. Our brains can go to great lengths to prove old stories true.

We keep trying to make the existing narrative true because that is a lot more comfortable than questioning a long-held belief. Like your loud uncle who is deeply entrenched in his political views at Thanksgiving dinner, your brain really wants to be right and looks for any and all evidence to support its case.

The good news is that your self-identity can change and evolve over time.

It's not what you look at that matters. It's what you see.
~Henry David Thoreau

The story you tell yourself leads to the actions you take, which creates your results. Disempowering stories lead to disappointing results.

So how do you rewrite the limiting beliefs you have into something that empowers you?

The first step is to uncover the limiting belief in the first place.

Author and speaker Jon Acuff talks about how old thought patterns are like broken soundtracks[17] in our brains. His advice for rooting out limiting beliefs is to write down a dream or a desire and listen to the reaction:

- What thoughts come up?
- Listen to your brain.
- Then ask yourself three questions.

Example:

"I want to lose weight so that I can get out there and start dating again."

Thoughts that come up:

"I can never lose weight for very long."

"Who would want to date me looking like this?"

"I hate diet food."

Then for each thought, ask yourself three questions.

1. Is it true?
2. Is it helpful? Does it move me forward or hold me back?
3. Is it kind? If I said it to a friend, would they still want to be my friend?

---

17 Soundtracks by Jon Acuff

Let's walk through this example.

"I can never lose weight for very long."

1. Is it true? *Maybe.*
    a. It's possible that you have a lot of evidence from the past that makes this thought feel really true.

2. Is it helpful? *No.* Does it move me forward or hold me back? *Holds me back.*
    a. Having a defeatist attitude is probably not going to help you feel motivated.

3. Is it kind? *No.* If I said it to a friend, would they still want to be my friend? *Not likely.*
    a. Can you imagine having coffee with a friend who tells you they are trying to lose weight and you tell them "Yeah, but you can never keep it off." I don't think you'd be friends for very long.

Two out of the three questions are "no". Therefore, this thought is a limiting belief.

"Who would want to date me looking like this?"

1. Is it true? *Who knows?*
    a. Though if you go on a date thinking *"Why would this guy or gal want to date me?"* that's probably not putting off the vibe that's going to attract the right person to you.

2. Is it helpful? *No.* Does it move me forward or hold me back? *Holds me back.*
    a. Your brain will always look to find answers to the questions you ask yourself. If you tell your brain to find the answer to *"Who would want to date me looking*

like this?" then your brain will filter for unhelpful answers.

3. Is it kind? *No.* If I said it to a friend, would they still want to be my friend? *Nope.*

    a. Saying that to a friend would be really hurtful.

Two and a half out of the three questions are "no". This thought is a limiting belief.

"I hate diet food."

1. Is it true? *Maybe.*

    a. There are probably some foods you don't like. That's natural. But there are a lot of foods out there. Have you really given yourself a chance to like them? How might you look for healthy foods that you do like?

2. Is it helpful? *No.* Does it move me forward or hold me back? *Holds me back.*

    a. Telling yourself that you hate diet food becomes a self-fulfilling prophecy and traps you in junk food hell.

3. Is it kind? *Not really.* If I said it to a friend, would they still want to be my friend? *Questionable.*

    a. Again, imagine having coffee with a friend who tells you they are trying to lose weight and you tell them "But you hate diet food!" You're shooting them down before they even get a chance to take off.

You're looking for three yeses. If they're not "yeses", then the thought is a limiting belief that is not helping you.

Another way to sniff out a limiting belief is that they often come attached to definitive words like "always" and "never."

For example:
- "I always overdo it when I go out with my friends."
- "I have no willpower when it comes to ice cream."
- "I'll never be able to go on vacation and enjoy what I eat again."

These words are a clue that your inner critic is talking and telling you a limiting belief.

Once you've sniffed out a limiting belief, remove the definitive word(s) and remove the context of weight loss. Then look for evidence of the opposite in your life outside the realm of diet and weight loss.

For example, let's say you have a limiting belief that says, *I'm never successful with weight loss because I always give up when I get frustrated by lack of progress.*

STEP 1: Remove the definitive word(s) and remove the context of weight loss.
- "I'm not successful because I give up when I get frustrated by lack of progress."

STEP 2: Look for examples of the opposite outside the realm of weight loss.
- The opposite of giving up is persevering. Especially in the face of setbacks or lack of progress.
- When in your life have you persevered despite setbacks or lack of progress?
  - Maybe in school?
  - Your family?
  - At work?

110

Julia felt like a complete failure when it came to weight loss. She'd tried to lose weight many times. And succeeded. But it always came back. She felt defeated and ready to give up again.

She told me, *"I always do this. I lose a few pounds, but then I lose steam. Life gets busy and I just get tired of working so hard to lose weight. So I give up."*

I asked her, *"Do you ALWAYS give up? Let's look outside the realm of weight loss. When is an example of a time that you persevered through something that was meaningful to you, but had its challenges?"*

It turned out she had put herself through nursing school while raising her daughter. Working, and going to school, and raising a child were a lot to juggle. They each certainly had their challenges. Yet she persevered and now enjoyed a meaningful career in nursing and her daughter was in high school.

I asked her what kind of character strengths it took for her to accomplish all of that. She said things like strength, courage, determination, not quitting even when it was hard. She already had what it took to keep going within her. She just needed to see it.

Have you earned a degree? Raised a child? Applied for a job? All of these are examples of things that are hard and require grit, perseverance, and resilience in the face of challenges, and little evidence of progress.

And yet, you persevered.

You probably have quite a few examples of times that you were successful because you decided not to give up, even when you were frustrated by a lack of progress. You clearly have those powerful character traits within you. They are there. If you're looking for it, there is evidence in your life that you are a strong, dedicated, resilient person capable of accomplishing really impressive things!

But you have to be looking for that evidence in order to find it.

When you focus on the reasons why you cannot achieve your goals, those obstacles loom large in your perception and crowd out the possibility of success.

Naturally, if you're constantly thinking about why you cannot succeed, that becomes a self-fulfilling prophecy.

Instead, how can you focus on the characteristics and strengths that would be necessary in order to achieve your goal? Then look into your past and find examples of how you've exhibited those characteristics before.

How can you pull those same character strengths into your weight loss efforts?

If you're struggling to find a time in the past when you exhibited those character strengths, then think into the future. Who would you have to become to be the kind of person who can achieve your goal? What's a small way you can live into who you want to become today?

Your brain looks to find evidence of what you're thinking. When you think a thought over and over again, it becomes more true because your brain filters for evidence of it. That evidence influences your actions, making that belief become a self-fulfilling prophecy.

Your thoughts are incredibly powerful. Choose yours wisely.

STEP 3: Ask Better Questions

When I first thought about writing this book, I thought, "Who would want to listen to me? Why would anyone read my book?"

As you might imagine, with such a helpful question in my mind, I procrastinated writing it....FOR SEVEN YEARS.

The brain is like a puzzle solving machine. Input a question, an answer comes out.

The quality of your questions determines your trajectory. If you ask yourself, "Who would want to date me looking like this?" then your brain is gonna come up with an answer. It's just that the answer isn't going to feel very good. Garbage in, garbage out.

In addition, big scary questions like, "How am I going to keep up this intense workout program?" makes your brain freak out and go into self-sabotaging mode.

Why not hack into your brain's natural puzzle solving programming with tiny, positive questions that (a) don't trigger warning bells in your subconscious mind and (b) get your brain looking for ways to help you achieve the things you want in life?

For example:

- "What's wrong with me? Why can't I have any willpower?"
  - Can become "What's one helpful choice I made for myself today?"
- "Why won't the scale go down?"
  - Can become "What is something I appreciate about my body no matter what the scale says?"
- "Why did I do this again? I always go overboard on Oreos!"

- ○ Can become "What's one little thing I learned from overeating last night?"
- • "How can I find time to meal plan when I'm so busy?"
  - ○ Can become "What can I do in five minutes a day to make me healthier?"

This allows the brain to focus on problem solving. Ask the question often enough, you'll find the brain turning it over to eventually come up with interesting solutions.

Try and get clear on what you're saying in your mind and see how you can tweak those disempowering questions into something small that opens up your mindset.

"Life isn't about finding yourself. Life is about creating yourself."
~*George Bernard Shaw*

TAKE IT FURTHER

Check out https://confidentbody.coach/book/ for a fillable worksheet on identifying and shifting limiting beliefs.

Are You a Sprinter or a Gardner?

Janeen had gone on a diet to lose weight for her daughter's wedding. She was seriously motivated to fit into her perfect dress and look amazing on her daughter's special day. And she did.

However, I didn't meet Janeen until seven months after her daughter's wedding when she'd gained back thirty-five of the forty pounds she had lost prior to the wedding.

Janeen created a goal for herself to reach a specific target weight in time for the wedding. She went on that diet like a runner sprinting toward the finish line with laser focus on the end goal.

But what happens when you reach the finish line? The very nature of a diet is that it's temporary. That temporary nature creates a hidden belief underneath that says you can "go back to normal" once you reach the finish line. The problem is, "normal" is what led to weight gain in the first place.

It is this kind of thinking that very predictably leads to the yo-yo dieting cycle of losing weight and gaining it back on.

How many diets have you tried in the past?

Keto? Paleo? Weight Watchers?

How many times have you lost weight, only to gain it back again?

All diets work to some extent.

The problem is that they don't teach you how to think about eating in a sustainable way. What they teach you is how to diet.

Diets don't address those underlying beliefs you have about yourself. Diets try to change you from the outside in. But REAL change happens from the inside out.

It's tempting to think of weight loss as something with a finish line. Once you reach your goal weight, you've won! Now you can rest.

But that mindset can backfire.

Real, lasting change happens when you focus on WHO you are becoming as a part of this process, rather than just the destination.

Try imagining it this way:

Think of your body weight and your health like a garden and you are the gardener.

You can get that garden looking gorgeous! Garden of the Month Club! However, if after that, you leave it alone and go back to old habits, what will happen?

The weeds will start to grow.

If you tend your garden regularly with love and care, it will stay beautiful.

Weeds will come up. That's nature. There's nothing wrong with you as a gardener if a weed crops up. The key is to pull those weeds and cultivate your garden on an ongoing basis rather than a big push with a finish line.

Habits Are Like Onions

Shrek[18]

For your information, there's a lot more to ogres than people think.

Donkey

Eegggzzzaaaample?

Shrek

Example? Okay, um… Ogres are like onions! (He holds out his onion.)

Donkey

(Sniffs the onion.) *They stink?*

---

18 Shrek, 2001 Dreamworks Entertainment

Shrek

Yes – – Noooo!

Donkey

They make you cry?

Shrek

No!

Donkey

You leave them in the sun, they get all brown, start sproutin' little white hairs?

Shrek

No!

Layers!

Onions have layers. Ogres have layers!

Onions have layers.

You get it? We both have layers.

(He heaves a sigh and then huffs and walks off.)

The movie *Shrek* has a special place in my heart. On our second date, my husband and I opted for a low-key movie night and rented Shrek from the Blockbuster video near my apartment. We popped the VHS cassette into the player and felt ourselves falling for each other, just like Shrek and Fiona. Awwww.

Turns out, this all-time great movie is more than just a love story. Who would've thought there'd be so much wisdom in a story about an ogre who just wants to live in his swamp in peace?

In the scene above, Shrek is trying to explain to Donkey that there's more to ogres than just destroying villages. People look at Shrek and judge him based on the scary ogre they see on the surface. But he wants more from life than that.

Habits can be the same way. We think we know how to change habits based on the actions we change on the surface. But there's a lot more to it than that.

For example: "I have to go to the gym today so I can rock a bikini this summer" is a very different message to your subconscious mind than "I go to the gym because I like how it makes me feel. I'm the kind of person who goes to the gym."

So let's imagine that habit change is like the layers of an onion.[19]

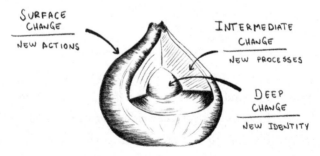

Surface Change: New actions

A simple change in behavior is the outside layer of the onion that gets crusty and kinda yellow sometimes. It's a surface level change.

---

19 Adapted from James Clear Identity Based Habits https://jamesclear.com/identity-based-habits

Just like the outer layer of the onion, surface level behavior change peels away and flakes off easily at the first sign of stress or a break in routine.

Most diets focus only on surface change.

Ex: "*For the next three weeks, I'm eating only chicken, kale, and vegetables.*"

These are the hardest to maintain because they have the least depth.

Intermediate Change: New processes

Peel back the layers a little and you get a change in process or how you do things.

Programs that focus on habit change can have a more lasting effect because they focus on the process, rather than the outcome.

Ex: "*Instead of figuring out what I'll eat in the moment, I'll create a system for meal planning every Sunday.*"

Changes you make in your processes are easier to maintain because they reduce the number of decisions you have to make in the moment.

Deep change: New identity

Deep change happens at the heart of the onion. How you see yourself has changed. You embody the identity of who you are becoming. The core of who you are looks different than it did before.

Ex: "*I go to the gym every day because I'm an athlete. Athletes work out.*"

Identity-based changes are the easiest to maintain because they are an extension of your beliefs about yourself.

When you incorporate the change into your identity, your behavior becomes about who you are becoming and the kind of person you want to be, rather than striving for some illusory finish line. It's not a one-time thing. It's a practice; a discipline.

> *"Improvements are only temporary until they become*
> *part of who you are."*
> *~James Clear*

Let's Get Muddy

I love mud runs. Must be something about my soccer goalie nature that likes to get dirty. I had done a few over the years. But then I heard about the Spartan Race. A mud run with obstacles? Whoaaaaaa! That seemed completely awesome and out of reach for me. I mean these people swing from ropes and jump over fire and you have to do like a million burpees if you mess up. I could never do that.

For years I told myself "Wouldn't that be cool to run a Spartan Race?" But I never signed up. Because of good old-fashioned FEAR. It scared the hell out of me. Could I actually finish a race like that? What if I failed? I had so much admiration for people who had done them and yet couldn't see myself in that same category.

Then one year, in a fit of New Year's resolution madness, I decided to go for it. I signed up and hit "confirm" on my registration.

I felt a moment of elation! Immediately followed by "Oh my God, what have I done?"

For the next five months, my workouts were fueled out of ⅓ motivation and ⅔ fear. The day of the race I was so nervous, I made my family get there two hours early. During the race, I just wanted to prove to myself that I could do it.

As it turned out, it was fun! I failed some obstacles miserably. And I completed some that I didn't expect to. The last obstacle required you to jump over a (small) line of logs that were on fire. I crossed the finish line and went straight to my husband and said, "We need to do this together."

For weeks after that race I was riding a high of confidence because I had blown my mind around what I believed I was capable of.

Sometimes when we're trying to make a new behavior into a habit, we focus on the action we're taking in order to get a specific result.

For example:

Action-Result based thinking:

- "I'll go to the gym today because I'm trying to lose weight."
- "I'll choose a salad at the restaurant because I'm on a diet."
- "I won't eat chocolate for the next 30 days because I'm doing a cleanse."

Action-Result based thinking requires a consistent replenishment of motivation and willpower. On the other hand, identity-based actions are a lot easier because they come from within.

Identity-Action based thinking:
- "I am an athlete and I exercise regularly to stay fit."
- "I'm a healthy eater and salad makes me feel good."
- "I'm in tune with my body. I avoid sugar because of how it impacts my hormones."

Running that Spartan race changed my identity.

Before it, I operated in action-result thinking. "I work out for the sole purpose of being able to complete the race." Afterward, I operated from identity-action thinking. "I am a Spartan racer. Spartans work out."

Your inner identity is the key to hacking your subconscious mind and making healthy choices your normal default behavior.

But short of jumping over a bunch of logs on fire, how do you magically go from where you are to who you want to be?

STEP 1: Start Where You're At

How do you currently see yourself?

Are you the kind of person who defaults to ordering fries when you go out unless you're "on a diet"? How do you eat on weekends when you're less strict with yourself? What sort of exercise do you like, if at all?

Any answer is okay! This is not about blame or shame. This is about being honest with yourself and knowing where you're starting from.

STEP 2: How would you LIKE to see yourself?

Future you sees herself or himself differently. Let's call her "Healthy You."

Take a second to imagine your future self. You've lost the weight you want to lose and you're living a whole new lifestyle. What does she eat on a regular basis? How often does she exercise?

More importantly, what does "Healthy You" believe about herself? How would she complete this sentence: "I am the kind of person who..."

STEP 3: Take it one thought at a time.

One small step at a time, proactively shift your thinking toward making your healthy habits a permanent part of your identity.

Little changes in how you see yourself in the moment lead to big transformation over time.

Let's look at "Old You" and "Healthy You" and put them both on a number line, each at one end.

Like let's imagine that "Old You" is -10.

0 is in the middle (neutral).

And "Healthy You" is +10.

No matter where you currently are on the number line, you don't have to choose to be either -10 or +10. There's a whole bunch of variations of choices and thoughts in between.

For example, let's say you're going to a cookout this weekend and there's plenty of less-than-healthy food choices.

How can you go from ... let's say a -9 choice to a -7 choice?

-10 Old You: "Well, my diet is ruined so I might as well eat whatever. So bring on the burgers and fries and beer and dessert."

-7 Old You: "I love burgers and fries. But I could probably skip the dessert."

<u>-1 Neutral You</u>: "I love me some fries, but I don't care that much about the bun. So I'll have my fries, but no bun. And just a small portion of dessert."

<u>+1 Neutral You</u>: "The desserts here aren't ones that are really worth the calories for me. So I'll skip that for now, and really enjoy a few fries because they taste better. And I'll skip the bun and add a few veggies from the veggie tray."

<u>+7 Healthy You</u>: "I really wish there was a salad here because burgers and fries make my stomach feel awful. There is a veggie tray. I'll fill up with that and maybe have a burger with no bun."

<u>+10 Healthy You</u>: "There's a veggie tray here. Plus there's lettuce to go on top of the burger patty. I can make a burger salad out of this and create some yummy goodness out of this!"

Basically, I'm saying you don't need to feel obligated to make the +10 choice all the time. And if you tried to, that might be a lot of pressure to put on yourself and it could lead to giving up.

Leveling up your choices from…

- not great to…
- maybe not amazing, but better to…
- neutral to…
- kind of okay to…
- pretty good…

….over time and consistently is how you go from "Old You" to "Healthy You."

Go On a Treasure Hunt

If you want to change your identity to the person you are becoming, first you need to know who you want to become. Then you need to train your brain to look for evidence to prove to yourself that you are becoming that person.

Think about your future self. Future you has gotten to where you want to go. Future you feels great and feels confident about being able to maintain their weight.

Complete this sentence: "Future me is the kind of person who..."

- What does future you think about themself?
- How does future you view food?
- How does future you eat / behave on weekends? On vacation? During the holidays?
- What are the things future you wants to eat? What are the things future you doesn't want to eat?
- When you notice a craving, ask yourself "What would my future self think about [X] food? Would they want it? What would future me be thinking at this moment?"

The more you can get your brain into thinking the way that future you thinks naturally, the faster and easier it will be to become future you.

Then get to work looking for examples of how you acted like future you in a little way today. An important part of the process of changing your identity is to internalize your successes.

Remember, the brain is always looking for evidence to prove its beliefs right. The identity you have now is based on the evidence you have from the past.

Little wins are like buried treasure that will accumulate into a treasure trove of beliefs. Make a big deal out of your small wins! Huge change is built on the back of tiny pieces of evidence, proving to your brain that you actually CAN become the person you want to be.

Little bits of proof are the breadcrumbs your subconscious mind needs to follow in order to buy into the person you are becoming. Train your brain to look for those treasures and pieces of proof with open ended questions.

- "What is an example of how I took good care of myself today?"
- "How did I show up for myself today?"
- "What is a tiny way that I am making progress?"

Give your brain a puzzle to solve in the form of an open-ended question and it will get to work finding the answer for you.

CHAPTER 7

HOW TO MAKE THE SCALE YOUR B****

When I was a kid, I put a Band-Aid on everything. Skin your knee?

Put a Band-Aid on it.

Rough up your elbow?

Put a Band-Aid on it.

Got a freckle?

Put a Band-Aid on it.

Wait. Is that an open patch of skin unprotected and vulnerable to the elements?

Put a Band-Aid on it.

I even once put a Band-Aid on my dresser drawer because it had a scratch on it.

Mom called me The Band-Aid Queen of 1978. (My first and only pageant title.)

My little three-year-old brain decided that a Band-Aid was the answer for everything. And that's fine for a three-year-old. (Though mom did get a little tired of running out of Band-Aids.)

But these days with diet culture, the scale can be seen as the answer to everything. And that can get you into trouble.

"To the man who only has a hammer,
everything he encounters begins to look like a nail."
~Abraham Maslow

When the scale is the only tool you're using to measure your weight loss progress, everything is either wonderful or terrible. There is no in-between.

I can walk up to the scale feeling pretty good about myself and even expecting to see some positive results. Then the number comes back and it's not what I expected. That one little number can ruin my whole day.

Why is it that a piece of plastic and metal that sits on the floor can have so much power over us?

The scale is a tool that produces data. It gives you a number. You know what else does that? A calculator.

Have you ever felt bad about yourself because of a number that showed up on the calculator screen?

Me neither.

But the scale is a different story. Why?

The problem is not the number itself. The number is neutral. The problem is what we make the number MEAN.

What are you making that number mean about you?

"What am I doing wrong! This always happens. I'll never lose weight."

When the scale doesn't tell you exactly what you want it to, you get frustrated. Over time, frustration can lead to giving up.

But it doesn't have to be that way.

First, let's put the scale in perspective.

The scale is a useful tool in the weight loss toolbox. But it's a bit of a blunt instrument. The number on the scale is not always directly correlated to what you're eating.

There are all sorts of things outside of your control that can make the scale go up temporarily.

Here are just a few examples of things that can make the scale go up that aren't "your fault":

- Hormone fluctuations
- An injury
  - Like a bruise that leads to swelling or recovering from a medical procedure.
- Lifting weights
  - Lifting weights causes micro tears in the muscle. The body heals and strengthens the muscle. But part of the healing process involves little bits of fluid and swelling to tend to the muscle.
- Salty food
- Foods high in starchy carbs
  - Especially bread, pasta, rice, and potatoes. They soak up water like a sponge in your body.
- Poor sleep last night
- Needing to have a bowel movement
- Even the weather

So it helps to keep the scale in the proper perspective.

Reality Is a Shipwreck Compared to Perfect Expectations

Not only is the scale a little fuzzy when it comes to exactly measuring your weight, but then there's the story in your head about what it's supposed to do. Whether we admit it to ourselves or not, we all have a countdown clock in our minds that tells us when we should expect to see results.

However, that countdown clock may or may not be based in reality.

Often, the reality of our progress does not align with our expectations. We think that we should be losing faster. We think that the scale should only go in one direction. We think that we're doing it wrong if the scale doesn't move down or (Heaven forbid) goes up.

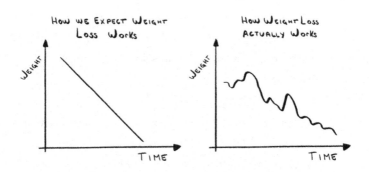

The way you feel about your progress is relative to your expectations.

Imagine I gave you $100. If you weren't expecting anything, you'd be thrilled! If you were expecting $1000, you'd feel ripped off. It's the exact same result. But different expectations create very different emotions.

Reality is a complete mess compared to perfect expectations.

The level to which you feel awesome or awful is relative to what your expectations are.

That's not to say that you shouldn't aim high! But there's nuance. Have high expectations of yourself in generalities and low expectations for specific events.

For example, let's say you're going to a barbeque this weekend. Have high expectations of how you can trust yourself, of knowing that you can tune into your body and listen to your fullness cues. But have low expectations on eating perfectly and avoiding every single fattening food that might be there.

Have high expectations of your progress over time, but low expectations from day to day or week to week.

Have high expectations of practicing your process (like meal planning or proactively choosing your thoughts) but low expectations of executing it perfectly.

Let's look at this from a different perspective.

Let's say you are a busy and successful professional. You've worked hard to build your business or your career to where it is over the course of the last several years.

Or perhaps you are a busy mom with a full family life. Maybe you're both!

You've worked hard to nurture your family and build your career over the course of the last several years. It's taken a lot of grit, patience, and determination to be at the place where you are now.

When you first started, what were your expectations for your career growth or family life? Were you expecting it to be linear and predictable? Always moving in a positive direction?

What was your career growth or family life actually like? My guess is that there were some successes and setbacks, ups and downs. Not every day was perfect. Yet you persevered, worked hard, and decided not to give up.

Why would you expect weight loss to go exactly as planned when basically nothing else in life does?

Weight loss is rarely a linear process. There are ups and downs, successes and setbacks. That is normal.

Expect it.

What if you could adopt the same mindset you use in your career or your family toward your weight loss journey?

Use Weight Loss Binoculars

When I was a kid, I was fascinated by how you could look through binoculars one way and they'd make what you're looking at seem much closer. Then flip them around and they make the thing you're looking at seem far away. (Okay, who am I kidding? I still think that's pretty cool.)

Human beings are motivated by progress, and it can be really frustrating when you don't feel like you're making the progress you want to. Long-term change takes time, and patience can be hard to come by when you're trying to lose weight.

When you're in the day to day of trying to lose weight, it can be tough to maintain perspective. So, use weight loss binoculars.

1) Zoom in: Make the next best choice.

   If you can keep your focus on the very short-term and simply concentrate on making the next best choice, then you're never more than one choice away from being right back on track.

2) Zoom out: Take the long view.

   Healthy weight loss is considered to be around one pound per week. If you were to take the total number of pounds you'd like to lose, and calculate a rate of one pound per week, what date on the calendar would that map out to? Then give yourself grace for the day-to-day fluctuations and keep the longer perspective in mind.

What A Middle School Science Fair Can Teach You About Weight Loss

Back in the day when I was a middle school science teacher, each year we would host a science fair. The students would need to come up with a project to demonstrate the scientific method. My favorite experiments were always the ones that dealt with plant growth because they were so straightforward and easy to see results.

- Ex: "What is the effect of fertilizer on plant growth?
- "What is the effect of different types of liquids (water, orange juice, apple juice) on plant growth?"

- "What is the effect of positive or negative thoughts on the growth of plants?"[20] (Yes, there's a real impact. Try it!)

The students would form a hypothesis, gather data, graph their results, and draw conclusions based on the data.

Often their hypothesis was correct. (It's not hard to guess that water is better for plant growth than orange juice.) But sometimes the results were surprising. Either way, they still made progress. Whether the hypothesis was correct or not, they always learned something.

What would it be like to treat your weight loss journey like a scientist?

Here's what I mean:

When a scientist conducts an experiment, they are constantly gathering data and forming conclusions.

If they form a hypothesis that turns out to be wrong based on the data, that does not mean they're a terrible scientist. They don't go around beating themselves up.

If a scientist treated their experiment the way we treat weight loss, they'd quit their research and pursue a career as a florist.

Instead, they view their results as simply information that helps them get closer to a more accurate conclusion from the data they've gathered. In fact, a negative hypothesis can be a wonderful discovery because it gets you (the scientist) one step closer to finding out what does work.

---

20 This is actually a real experiment from the book E Squared by Pam Grout. Spoiler: Positive thoughts helped the plants grow more. I've actually tried it. It works!

Of the 200 light bulbs that didn't work, every failure told me
something that I was able to incorporate into the next attempt.
~Thomas Edison

If we take that to the idea of weight loss....

- The number on the scale is data.
- What you eat is data.
- Your thoughts and feelings before emotional eating are data.
- What happened earlier in the day or week before binging on ice cream is data.
- Feeling gross after having five slices of pizza is data.
- Not sleeping well when you eat a bunch of sugary treats before bed is data.
- Your thoughts are data.

How might you look at those events with curiosity and try to learn a little about yourself and your thoughts? How might you use that information to help you have more knowledge and be more prepared the next time you're faced with a similar situation?

It's All Relative

I like to get up and exercise in the morning. It's not that I have amazing willpower. It's that I know I WON'T have the willpower or energy to do it later. So I get it out of the way before I'm awake enough to object.

Occasionally, my husband will stay in bed and work out later. (He's more disciplined later in the day than I am.)

On mornings when it's chilly in the house, he'll turn up the heat while I'm outside exercising. When I come back inside, it feels sooooo hot to me. Of course, I immediately go to the thermostat and turn it down. If I'm not sneaky enough and he sees me he'll say, "Stop turning down the heat! It's freezing in here!"

We are in the same house. The temperature is the same for both of us. But I'm hot and he's freezing. How do we know how we feel?

What if I walked into the warm house after I'm all hot and sweaty and said, "Hmmm, the temperature on the thermostat says 69. I guess I must be cold."

No! That's ridiculous!

Looking at the scale to tell you how you feel is like looking at the thermostat in the house to decide if you're hot or cold.

The thermostat measures the temperature in the house. It does not tell you how you feel.

The scale measures the mass of your body compared to the gravitational pull of the Earth. It does not tell you how you feel. You get to make the number mean anything you want. And you get to decide how you want to feel about yourself.

If you recognize that the scale tends to get in your head, try this:

→ Decide how you feel about yourself BEFORE you step on the scale.

You weigh the exact same amount before you step on the scale as you will 30 seconds later after the scale registers a number.

Decide ahead of time who determines the quality of your day, how you feel about yourself, or your worth. You or the scale?

You can choose ahead of time to tell yourself that "No matter what the scale says, I am choosing to see myself for the miraculous creation I am. Not 100% perfect and not 100% awful. There's a lot that I love about me, and this number is just data that can help inform my decisions, but it won't inform my opinion of me."

If you decide to get on the scale (totally optional), how might you decide AHEAD of time how you're going to feel about yourself?

When The Scale Goes Up for No Reason

"Ok Lizzie, that's great. But this morning I stepped on the scale, and I was up a lot. What the heck? How did I gain three pounds overnight?"

Deep breath.

As much as the scale is simply one tool to use and you get to decide how you feel about yourself, it still can be a useful tool for weight loss. And we have a lot of years of practicing looking to the scale to determine how we feel (or avoiding the scale to not think about it.) So it's pretty normal to still be miffed if the scale goes up.

Relax.

There's a good chance it's water weight.

Often when the scale goes up unexpectedly, that is telling you more about WHAT you ate yesterday rather than HOW MUCH. Specifically salt and carb-heavy foods.

Foods that have a high salt content or starchy carbs (like pasta, breads, rice, potatoes, crackers, etc.) will soak up water in your system and result in a higher number on the scale the next day.

150g of carbohydrates converts to about one pound of water (because it takes 3-5g of water to convert carbs to glycogen).

In terms of salt, it takes four cups of water to balance out about 400mg of sodium in the body. That roughly equals out to about two pounds of water.

CARBS + SALT

150g carbs ~ 1lb water

400mg sodium ~ 2lb water

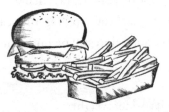

	carbs	sodium
1/4 lb hamburger —	0g	250 mg
+ bun	36g	320 mg
+ fries	28g	370 mg
	64g	940 mg

EQUATES TO .4lb + 4.7lb = 5.1 lb
OF WATER

If you've ever tried a low carb diet, you may notice that you're more likely to need to use the restroom during the night because your body is better at flushing out water with fewer carbs in your system.

> PRO TIP: If you're aiming to look slimmer for a specific event like a wedding, one hack you can use is avoid starchy or salty foods, particularly one to two weeks prior to the event.

> Because foods like bread, rice, pasta, potatoes, and flour products (like crackers and pretzels) soak up water, they can end up making you look or feel a little puffy.

> So avoiding them lets your body lean out a bit.

That doesn't mean that high starch or salty foods are bad. It just explains what you're seeing on the scale.

As you get back to your healthy habits, water retention will even itself out. Drinking lots of water will help your kidneys to flush things out as well. However, if you notice that you consistently have foods like pasta, rice, potatoes, bread, or salty foods in your diet, then it's gonna be hard to lose weight long term.

NOTE: If you're thinking, "Oh great. Now I have to cut out carbs altogether." Stop.

I would NOT suggest going cold turkey and eliminating foods you love altogether.

That just leads to feeling deprived. Feeling deprived leads to feeling like you're "on a diet." And feeling like you're "on a diet" suggests to your subconscious mind that one day you'll be "off" your diet.

Whatever actions you take to lose the weight are the same actions it will take to keep the weight off. So don't do anything drastic you can't see yourself doing 5 years from now.

However, if you DO want to look into reducing some of those foods gradually, here's a suggestion.

If you were to look at those food types (bread, rice, pasta, flour products like crackers & pretzels), which type of food would you miss the least?

Then, since you won't miss that as much, maybe aim to have one to two fewer servings of that type of food this week and see how you feel. Keep everything else the same for now.

In two weeks, assess and see how you're feeling. If you feel ready to reduce something else, great. If not, keep things as they are. 1% changes add up over time!

The Pesky Plateau

And then there are plateaus. Ugh.

They can be so frustrating.

You're logging the meals, you're eating the veggies, you're getting in some movement, and yet...the *bleeping* scale either stays the same or you gain and lose the same three pounds over and over again.

First, let's get real on what a true plateau actually is.

A true plateau is when your weight stays the same (within two to three pounds) for more than two weeks. So when your weight is mostly the same for four days in a row, try to be patient. Your body may be adjusting and recalibrating in ways that are not measured by the scale.

Also, let's get clear on expectations.

Plateaus are NORMAL.

Imagine you're driving across town to get to the hardware store.

Along the way, you stop at an intersection for a red light.

Your brain does not say, *"Oh no! We're off track! We've failed to get to the hardware store!"* because you know that stopping at a red light is just something that happens sometimes on the way to your destination.

You can look at a plateau or a stall or even an uptick of a few pounds in the same way.

What if you looked ahead at your weight loss journey and EXPECTED there to be a plateau or two in there somewhere? "Oh hello plateau. I've been expecting you." How would that change your mindset?

Plateaus are normal because the body is really good at adjusting and trying to keep things at equilibrium. Losing weight goes against the grain of what the body wants to do. A plateau is just your body doing its job effectively. It's okay.

Here's some science behind plateaus:
- Total Daily Energy Expenditure (TDEE):
  - The amount of calories you burn in a day is called your total daily energy expenditure (TDEE).
- Basal Metabolic Rate (BMR):
  - When you lose weight, your basal metabolic rate (BMR) decreases, therefore lowering your overall TDEE.
- Metabolic adaptation:

- ○ Your body realizes that you are feeding it fewer calories than normal, so it becomes more efficient at using calories (Uhm, thanks?)
- Adaptive Thermogenesis:
  - ○ Your TDEE goes down as your body becomes more efficient. (Basically your body slows down your metabolism to avoid starvation.)

As you get closer to your body's ideal weight, it becomes harder to keep losing weight because

a) your body is smaller so it needs fewer calories

and

b) your body is getting increasingly efficient at storing away calories for a rainy day.

Sometimes your ideas around what is a normal portion size are the same as they used to be when you were at a higher weight.

You're comparing how much food it takes to maintain a lower weight to what you used to eat at a heavier weight. It feels like a lot less food! While it seems obvious that you'd put less fuel into a compact car than into an SUV, it's not so obvious when you're thinking about the fact that your smaller body now needs less fuel.

One of the greatest motivators to the human mind is progress. Making a lot of effort and seeing little progress can be a recipe for frustration.

Rather than getting frustrated by a plateau, try to get busy on solving it.

When a plateau happens, there are a couple of things you can do.

1. Look at the big picture. How far have you come already? Give yourself credit and celebrate what you've already accomplished.

2. Manage your mindset. If the scale is getting under your skin, stop using it for a few days. Tune into your body and see how you feel.

3. Be patient. Lack of weight loss for a period of two to three weeks does not mean that anything is wrong. It means your body is adapting and adjusting.

4. Don't give up. If you go back to old habits, you'll gain weight.

5. Look for other ways to measure progress beyond the scale. I've known folks who've gone down two clothing sizes before the scale moved. The body can change in a lot of ways. How do your clothes fit? How's your sleep or energy lately? How do you feel in your body? If the scale did not exist, how would you feel about your progress?

6. To break a plateau, try and mix things up a bit. Eat your meals earlier. Add more protein. Try fewer carbs. Eat dessert at three p.m. instead of eight p.m. Do a bunch of experiments and see what happens. Treat it lightly.

7. Move more during the day. Non-exercise activity thermogenesis (NEAT) makes up 15% of your total calorie burn. NEAT is not a specific exercise (like time on the peloton.) NEAT is the kind of movement you do during the day, like standing up from your desk two to three times per hour and moving around the house or

office. Pick things up and put them down. Go upstairs and come back down. etc.

8. Consider a small increase in healthy calories one day a week.

   a. Give your body a gentle reminder that there's no famine and eat a little more on one day. Just make it as healthy as you can and try not to go overboard.

9. Try experimenting with smaller portions for a week or two. It's easier to treat a small change lightly in the brain when you think of it like, "Let's just experiment for a little while and see what happens."

Remember, if you simply keep going, reaching your goal is inevitable.

Don't give up. You've got this!

Change the Metric

One time in high school, some friends of mine and I decided to make cookies at a sleepover. Since there were four of us, we divided up the tasks of measuring out the butter, flour, salt, baking soda, etc. We mixed up all the ingredients, tossed them in the oven and waited eagerly for the cookies to come out (after several spoonfuls of dough, of course.)

However, when the cookies came out, they didn't look right. They were kinda runny and burned. "What happened?" As we investigated, we realized that whoever was in charge of the flour put in 1 ½ cups of flour instead of 2 ½ cups. The process of making the cookies definitely impacted the result.

We live in an outcome focused culture. It's human nature to want to see results from our efforts. However, we often forget that the results are the outcome of whatever process we used to get there. Focusing only on the scale is like making cookies without paying attention to how much flour you put in the mix.

Focusing only on results leads to perfectionism. Perfectionists need positive results to motivate them to go through the process. It's like having blind hope that finally THIS time this diet will work. When those results don't show up as fast as you expected, it feels demoralizing and can lead to giving up too early.

If the scale is getting into your head, perhaps it makes sense to remove it from the equation for a little while.

Here's the thing: the scale measures a RESULT, not actions.

When you measure your progress by the scale, you're looking at an end product that is not completely within your control. Let's say you have an injury, and your body has inflammation. The scale goes up. Let's say your hormones are in their natural cycle and that is causing some water retention. The scale goes up. There are many reasons why the scale may not behave the way you expect. Some of those reasons are within your control, but not all of them.

By using the scale as your only and ultimate measure of success, you're gambling your feeling of success and the positive rewards you get from seeing progress on something that is not 100% within your control.

First, identify the actions that create the results you're looking for. Then measure your progress based on the positive actions you're taking.

It is those actions that will ultimately create the results you want. When you only focus on results, it can get discouraging. Sometimes you can even stop doing those positive actions because you feel demoralized. That, of course, then guarantees a negative result.

So change the metric.

If you can shift your focus to feeling proud of yourself for the very real and tangible positive actions you've been taking, then you can cultivate positive emotions that help you maintain progress.

Here are some ways to measure your success based on actions that ARE within your control.

- Exercise:
  - Number of minutes walked per day or week
  - Number of consecutive days of stretching
- Nutrition:
  - Number of days eating a veggie as a snack
  - Number of consecutive days without eating after seven p.m.
- Portion Control:
  - Number of meals eating on a smaller plate
- Mindfulness:
  - Number of times you put the fork down during the meal
- Reducing the amount of something:
  - Number of days I only had X amount of Y

Do you sometimes have a hard time giving yourself credit for how much progress you've made? Is your eye on the prize, instead of the little things you're doing consistently every day? It can be so easy to not even see the progress you've made because you are so focused on where you're not.

Progress comes from owning the actions you've been taking. Because it is in those actions that you are becoming the kind of person who can build the future you're driving toward.

There are so many things you can measure to track your success that are WITHIN your control. Bank your progress on the tangible ways that you are positively changing your life and the results will take care of themselves.

What's The Whole Point Anyway?

The whole point of this journey is not about hitting a number on the scale. You may get sidetracked by the number on the scale, but it's not what you're after.

The reason why we pursue any goal is because of how we think it will make us FEEL. A person doesn't buy a fancy car for the car itself. They buy the car for how they think they will feel when driving it or how owning it will make them feel about themselves.

Weight loss is no different.

Most of the time, the reason why folks want to lose weight is because they think it will make them feel confident or healthier or sexy or worthy or enough.

It all comes down to how you FEEL.

You can do all of that without ever looking at the scale. The scale does not measure your level of confidence or how much energy you have. The scale doesn't tell you how happy you are, nor does it measure your ability to have a good day. The scale doesn't measure your sexiness or worthiness.

YOU get to decide all of that.

What would it be like to let go of what you're making the number on the scale mean to you?

Let's do a thought experiment.

Though this is unlikely, let's say that you don't lose any weight (or any more weight).

Scenario A:

You don't lose any more weight and decide to give up. You go back to eating mindlessly or even punishing yourself with food.

Where are you five years from now?

Scenario B:

You don't lose any more weight. However, you begin to notice how your body feels when you eat salads for lunch and more fruits and veggies in general.

You start to sleep better and have more energy. You just FEEL better. The foods you used to eat make you feel bloated, sluggish, and kinda gross.

So you decide that most of the time, you'd rather have the healthier food, because it just FEELS better.

Where are you five years from now?

Scenario C:

You don't lose any more weight. However, you do a lot of work on your relationship with your body, and you begin to learn to appreciate yourself and your body.

You take time to proactively look for what's right about you. You feel like you have a partnership with your body, and you realize that your body is the vehicle through which you get to experience everything this life has to offer.

Where are you five years from now?

In all three of those scenarios, you are the exact weight you are now. But the outcomes are different.

What is this journey REALLY about for you?

If it's only about hitting a number on the scale, you can get there and still not be happy.

Sometimes the heaviest things you have to lose are your thoughts about yourself.

When we try to hurry up weight loss based on our own timeline, we miss the most important part of rebuilding our relationship with ourselves.

The scale can be a useful tool on your weight loss journey, but not if it's going to wreck your mindset.

Your mindset is your most powerful asset.

What if the number on the scale was just neutral data that's telling you something about your experiment?

What Are You Waiting For?

Janelle is a wife, a mom, a business owner, and an altogether amazing human.

But she was feeling FRUS-TRA-TED!

"Everything feels so hard. I feel like I'm pushing all the time to exercise or avoid sugar. And God forbid, don't eat bread!"

I asked her, "What's this all for? How do you want to FEEL in your body?"

She said things like:

- Capable
- Strong
- Flexible
- Beautiful

I said, "Okay, what is an example of something you did today in which your body was capable of completing it?" (Like getting a cup of coffee.)

"What's an example today when you were strong enough to do something?" (Like open the drawer to get a shirt.)

"What's an example of when you were flexible today?" (Maybe bending down to tie your shoes?)

"What's an example of one thing that makes you feel beautiful?" (Ex: I really like my eyes.)

So often I see clients stuck in the belief that they will feel better or proud or whatever once they lose weight. They don't think they can access those feelings now.

That belief creates so much suffering.

Why wait to feel good?

===> The key is to identify what FEELING is it that you want to FEEL.

And then get to work looking for evidence of that in your life already.

The more you can bring that FEELING into the present, the more your future becomes your reality.

You do not have to wait to enjoy your life based on what the scale says.

You don't need to weigh a certain amount or be a certain jeans size in order to feel the way you want to feel about yourself. Look for evidence today.

CHAPTER 8
HOW TO HANDLE
SELF-SABOTAGY THOUGHTS

How Crocodiles Explain Self Sabotage

While deployments are certainly no fun, one of the perks of being a military family is that you get to travel and see some different parts of the world. In 2014 we were stationed in Guam for about a year. Guam is actually not that far from Australia, so we decided to visit.

Australia has a surprising number of animals that can kill you. So naturally, we needed to check them out. We drove an hour and a half on the left side of the road up a tight, winding, coastal highway to visit Hartley's Crocodile Adventures. What a place!

There was one exhibit that had seating where you could watch the "show." We arrived before the show began so there wasn't much to see. Just a murky pond with a fence around it. So far, I wasn't impressed.

Then the gamekeeper came out and started telling us about Hagrid, the croc that lived in this pond. "Really?" I thought. The pond didn't look very deep. I didn't know where a supposedly 16-foot crocodile would be hiding.

And then he got out a pole with a piece of chicken meat tied to the end and dangled it over the pond. In half a second, the water erupted. A massive animal burst up to snatch the meat and then disappeared. Not even half of its body was out of the water and even just the part I could see was larger than the gamekeeper.

Google "Hartley's Crocodile Adventures Hagrid" images and you'll see what I mean.

Self-sabotage can be just like Hagrid lurking hidden beneath the surface of the pond. We don't realize it, but there can be old limiting stories tucked away beneath the surface of our conscious awareness, waiting to pop out and sabotage our success.

It might seem strange to think that there's part of you that wants to stop your progress. But there are actually a number of reasons why someone might sabotage their efforts.

At its core, self-sabotage happens when there is inner conflict between a part of you that wants to lose weight and a part of you that doesn't.

> *"Whoa, whoa, whoa. I can confidently say that*
> *100% of me wants to lose weight."*

I get that!

But that's your conscious mind speaking.

Sometimes there is a different story lurking underneath the murky waters of your awareness.

It can be frustrating to feel an involuntary craving for treats or to go off plan if you don't understand the mechanisms going on in your brain. It may make you wonder, "Where is this coming from? Why do I feel out of control? Why did I eat so much more than I planned?"

Nothing is taking over you and there is nothing wrong with you. Actually, self-sabotage is evidence that your brain is doing exactly what it is designed to do. Your brain is protecting you.

You are not broken.

Every successful weight loss story has self-sabotage in it.

Even the apostle Paul struggled with self-sabotage!

"What I don't understand about myself is that I decide one way, but then act another, doing things I absolutely despise...I can will it, but I can't do it. I decide to do good, but I don't really do it. I decide not to do bad, but then I do it anyway....Parts of me covertly rebel and just when I least expect it, they take charge."
~ Romans 7:15-23 Msg

We need to normalize self-sabotage before we can get past it. If you have a human brain, there is always some capacity for self-sabotage. It's not your fault!

SELF-SABOTAGE IS NORMAL.

Four Kinds of Croc-y Thoughts

When our son was in kindergarten, I came in and volunteered in the classroom from time to time. Their teacher, Ms. Tracy was a delightful, older lady who had A LOT more patience for the twelve little darlings in her class than I did.

155

One day, a boy named Dalton came up to me and said, "Ms. Lizzie, you're taller than Ms. Tracy. Does that mean you're older than her too?"

Dalton knew that the taller people in his life were the grown-ups. And he was taller than his younger sister too. So his little six-year-old brain came to the conclusion that if one person is taller than the other, that means they're older.

Makes sense to a six-year-old. It just doesn't happen to be true.

The same thing happens in our brains when our subconscious mind draws a conclusion that makes sense at the time but ends up resulting in a lot of our self-sabotage behavior.

Whatever limiting belief that might be at the root of your self-sabotage came from your brain trying to protect you in a way that made sense at the time. But now it's like Hagrid the croc, lurking beneath the surface of our awareness, waiting to pounce on your success.

When you're able to unravel some of those faulty subconscious conclusions, you can learn some interesting reasons why your subconscious mind might look at food as safety or comfort.

I've seen many examples of how an experience when a person was young turned into self-sabotaging behavior in the present.

Our psyches can create all sorts of coping mechanisms to help us deal with the things we experience. Over time, these coping mechanisms evolve into limiting beliefs.

I've had clients who:

- Were made fun of in school. So they learned to never eat in front of others and then binged when they got home.

- Had strict food restrictions as a child. They learned to eat in secret and to eat the Halloween candy all at once because they knew they wouldn't get it any other time of year.
- Were the victim of an assault. So they learned to protect themselves and hide behind a layer of fat so as not to be seen by a potential attacker.
- Saw someone they cared about suffer from an eating disorder. They learned that obsessing about food leads to pain, so they refused to be aware of what they ate to avoid being obsessed.
- Felt neglected by a mom who was hustling to be skinny to gain the attention of men. They learned that skinniness equals lovability. But since they didn't feel loved, that meant they shouldn't be skinny.
- Grew up with financial struggles and food was not always available. They learned to eat all they could when food was around because they never knew when it would run out.

All of these rationalizations happened beneath my clients' conscious awareness. On the surface, they'd tried all sorts of things to lose weight. But when we dove deeper, we were able to see why part of their subconscious mind wanted to resist losing weight.

> *"Resilience is often a slow unfolding of understanding.*
> *What did that experience mean to me?*
> *What were the gremlins mumbling?*

*Not only do we need to own our own story and love ourselves
in the process, we have to figure out the real story.
We also have to learn how to protect ourselves from shame
if we want to develop worthiness."*
~Brene Brown

Our brains are really great at protecting us. However, that can really create a challenge when it leads to behaviors that are hard to understand. We feel guilt and shame about our protective, self-sabotaging eating patterns when we don't understand what's underneath that behavior.

Limiting beliefs generally fall into one of four categories.

1. Low Self-Esteem
2. Fear of Failure
3. Fear of Change
4. Fear of Success

1) Low Self-Esteem

Sometimes, deep down, there can be a voice that says, "I don't deserve to succeed."

Maybe you experienced something difficult in the past that makes you feel like you're not worthy. Maybe you learned messages when you were young from grown-ups in your life that made you believe that you don't get to be happy.

Over time, that thought becomes a limiting belief that acts like the hardware in the wiring of a computer.

- Do you have a hard time accepting compliments?
- Do you feel like you hide your true self in order to please and gain approval from others?

- Do you immediately blame yourself for any slip-ups or perceived failures?

When you feel bad about yourself, it's easy to turn to food to feel better.

If your subconscious mind is operating on the underlying program of "I don't deserve success" or "I am unlovable" then you may find yourself doing inexplicable behaviors.

On the surface, you're consciously trying to achieve your goals! But if you look at it from the perspective of the subconscious mind, you're simply following the program that says, "I don't deserve to feel good." So you act accordingly by harpooning your success.

If you were taught to believe that you are "less than" when you were younger, that can be hard to overcome. It's not your fault if you were raised with certain expectations and beliefs around who you "should" be or what you're "supposed" to do.

However, you are RESPONSIBLE for it.

Once you recognize that these beliefs were put on you from someone or somewhere else, now you need to decide if you want to OWN them as your own. Or decide which beliefs and expectations you want to have for yourself and own those instead.

You get to choose what is true for YOU.

2) Fear of Failure

"What if I can't do it? I've tried losing weight so many times before. It might have worked a little, but I always gained it back. What if this time is just like all the others?"

159

Let's be honest. Failure hurts. Weight loss really impacts your identity and your primal sense of security and safety. The risk of failing at something so important can be scary.

If you're afraid of failing, (I mean, who isn't on some level?) it can be comforting to your subconscious mind to feel in control of that "failure" by sabotaging your efforts.

You avoid failing by not really trying.

For example, I might tell myself, "I'm not in the right head-space to lose weight right now." This protects my sense of self because if I really went all out and didn't succeed, that's failing. That HURTS.

But if I didn't totally try, then failing can't really be blamed on ME. It was my circumstances! So I get out ahead of the failure by not really trying and avoid that threat to my identity.

> *"It's not the literal consequences of failure that scare us.*
> *It is the fear that we'd fail at something that matters to us.*
> *It's not the failure we fear.*
> *It is what the failure means about who we are."*
> *~Stephen Guise[21]*

Often fear of failure gets dressed up and masquerades as per-fectionism. The subconscious loves perfectionism because it can hide there and hang out safely in the nice cool shadow of that boulder called Perfection. If the standard I'm aiming for is per-fection, then trying to meet it seems futile. It's easier to not try. Perfectionism is really a form of self-protection.

---

21 How To Be An Imperfectionist by Stephen Guise

I don't know about you, but I feel some version of fear several times a day.

Usually, I'm all wrapped up in the story in my head. However, when I can notice fear, I try to remind myself that fear is a sign that my ego is talking. My small self. The "me" that is rooted in my identity as it is in this minute.

I know that there is a deeper part of me that is not afraid. The wisp of the Divine that is in each of us whispers, "You are stronger than you think."

Fear is born from the little me. The lower case "I am."

When I can connect with the deeper "I AM," all there is is love.

"The arrival of fear isn't failure.
The arrival of fear is an invitation to bravery."
~Jon Acuff

3) Fear of Change

"I'm worried that I'll never be able to eat my favorite foods again, and I'll always feel deprived."
"My partner loves good food, and I don't want to give that up."
"I like to go out and have drinks with friends."

The subconscious mind views change as a massive threat. Think about it. Back on the savanna, if something was different (change) that could have meant a predator was nearby or a famine was coming. The primitive brain learned that change is BAD.

Changing your lifestyle, changing the way you look, and changing the way you see yourself can be a huge identity shift.

Guess what the subconscious mind thinks about that? It says *"Uh, no thank you. I'll pass. My job is to keep us safe. Change is not safe."*

Consciously, you may feel miserable at a higher weight. Subconsciously, your mind feels nice and cozy and safe there. From the perspective of the subconscious mind, it prefers the "devil you know" vs. "the devil you don't know" every day of the week and twice on Sunday.

It's natural to fear change. But when that comes to changing your habits to become healthier, it can seem like your brain is working against you (because it literally is.)

4) Fear of Success

"Why would I ever be afraid of achieving the thing I am working toward?"

Actually, lots of reasons.

For starters, success can be scary. When everything goes really well, everything changes. Sure, your body changes and your wardrobe changes. Those are nice changes. But also, your relationships change. The way you live your life and go out and interact with the world changes.

These more subtle changes can give your subconscious mind pause like, "Hey, I'm not totally 110% sure I really WANT this."

- *"What if I lose all the weight and I don't love my body? What if it doesn't look like I thought it would?"*
- *"If I lose weight, I'll get attention. I'll have to date." (Or "I'll no longer have a great excuse NOT to put myself out there.")*
  - It can be terrifying to be vulnerable in that way.

162

- Some of us have a story in our heads that says, *"Once I lose the weight I will finally...get my real estate license; start my YouTube channel;* [insert scary but ultimately challenging and rewarding project here]"
  - Losing weight means you no longer have a reason to NOT go for your dreams.
- Maybe you'll have to change your lifestyle and you're afraid you'll miss going out with the girls on Fridays.
- Maybe you'll lose some friends because you no longer keep the same habits they do.
- Maybe you'll start attracting what feels like unwanted attention.

Extra weight is a subconscious form of protection.

When we're overweight, we tend to be overlooked. Not seen. To be seen can be vulnerable. It is safe to play small.

Losing weight means that you risk being SEEN.

Every time you have success, that fear voice pipes up. You subconsciously start figuring out how to NOT have as much success so that you don't have to face the fear of what lies on the other side of success.

How Did a Reptile Get In My Brain?

You already know that there are two parts of your brain: the conscious mind (the prefrontal cortex where rational decisions get made) and the subconscious mind (where the brain puts things that can be done on auto-pilot).

The prefrontal cortex uses up **a lot of energy**, so the brain doesn't want to use it as much. Because the brain wants to save energy, it is always on the lookout for patterns that it can delegate to the subconscious mind.

Anything you do on repeat, whether it's good for you or not, gets delegated to the subconscious mind as a habit.

Over time, your brain has stored lots of things in your subconscious mind.

- Thoughts about food, your weight, and your abilities.
- Stuff you were told as a kid, like "Clean your plate."
- Rules around food from past diets.
- Opinions about yourself based on the opinions and judgments from others.
- Societal messaging from magazines and social media.

You have roughly 60,000 thoughts a day. Ninety-five percent of them are driven by the subconscious mind.

That's 57,000 thoughts a day that impact you, but you don't even know they're there.

That's why it's so important to take that five percent of thoughts you DO hear, and proactively program them on purpose.

The skill of undoing self-sabotage is recognizing that your proactive thoughts are the key to rewiring the thoughts you'll never hear because they're beneath your awareness.

This is why there is such a big difference between knowing what to do and actually doing it.

Knowing WHAT to do is stored in that five percent of conscious thought. Actually DOING IT comes from the ninety-five percent of those thoughts that are flying under the radar.

But that's not all.

Your brain likes to prove itself right. If those old stories from your subconscious mind are the only dialogue in your brain, then the RAS will filter for evidence to prove your stories right and filter out any evidence that could contradict the old stories.

Ex: Your brain may be filtering for examples of how you've not stayed on your plan in the past and filtered out all the positive choices you've been making. So it feels like you're messing up all the time because that is what your brain is telling itself to remember.

When you add judgment and shame to the mix, you get stuck in a downward spiral rather than moving toward solving things.

When you know how to notice an old thought and recognize it, then you can retool it.

"My experience is what I agree to attend to.
Only those items which I notice shape my mind."
~William James

How To Be a Crocodile Hunter

Steve Iwrin, the beloved "Crocodile Hunter," was famous for chasing down all kinds of dangerous animals, including big saltwater crocs. Before he passed away in 2006, he dedicated his life to finding crocodiles, learning more about them, and when necessary, relocating them to his conservation wildlife park in Australia.

He knew that while crocodiles can be dangerous, they were a natural part of our world and worthy of being respected, rather than hunted and destroyed.

In the same way, your self-sabotagy thoughts can be challenging. But they are not something you need to forcibly make go away. You can't!

Instead, you just need to be aware that they are there, spot them when they pop up, and redirect them when you can.

Fear of failure, change, success, etc. are totally normal human emotions. That's just your brain trying to protect you. It's doing its job!

There's nothing wrong with you when your brain offers up thoughts that have some flavor of "What if I fail?"

The more important thing to focus on is "What do I do about it?"

First, it's imperative to try and let go of guilt and shame. Those feelings only keep you in the downward spiral of self-sabotage.

Second, you've got to change the filter. You want your brain to be filtering for evidence that it IS working, and you ARE making positive choices.

Think of it like this:

There are some things you decide to spend money on in a conscious, proactive way. You make a conscious decision to buy a piece of furniture, a piece of clothing, or a kitchen appliance. And there are other things that you've set up on auto-payment like internet, your car payment, or a streaming service (Netflix anyone?)

The limiting belief in your subconscious mind is like the auto-payment for some old random subscription you got years ago and completely forgot about. It's drawing money out of your account each month, but you're not aware of it because you forgot about it, and you just haven't looked closely at your bank statement lately.

It's easy to let it keep going, because it's on auto-pay. You don't have to do a thing!

In order to change the auto-payment, it takes **AWARENESS**. You've got to dig into your bank statement and find out what's there. Next, you've got to hunt down the phone number or support email address of the company that is drafting your auto-payment.

Then you've got to actually send the email or make the phone call to the company and ask them to cancel your account. You're **REDIRECTING** what happens with the money.

Now imagine that the company said, "Okay, you can cancel your account. But in order to do so, you need to call us every day for six months. Every time you call, we'll reduce your payment a little bit so that by the end of the six months, your payment will be zero. But until then, you've got to demonstrate that you want a new pattern by putting in the effort." That takes effort and **PRACTICE**.

Your old self-sabotaging habits and thought patterns are the same way.

The outcomes we get in our life are a direct result of our thinking. You can go on a diet and change your behaviors temporarily. But if you never address the limiting beliefs underneath, you'll always end up getting the same results over time.

Past diets may have failed because you didn't know how to get to the root of your self-sabotaging behavior and change it at its source.

Now you can.

STEP 1: AWARENESS

To interrupt the pattern of self-sabotage, you need to identify the root of why you're sabotaging yourself. You've got to get clear on those old thoughts and patterns that are hidden in the recesses of your brain, operating on autopilot without your awareness.

How do you find that out?

1. Every time you have a slip up, overeat, or off-plan moment, stop and reflect. What happened? What triggered you to change your plan and do something different? The old thought pattern is hiding in the slip-ups, waiting for you to find it.

2. Write down what the trigger was. Here are some common ones:
   ○ Stress, like a long day at work.
   ○ Boredom.
   ○ Depriving yourself.
   ○ A stressful encounter "My mother-in-law called." "My boss criticized me."
   ○ Lack of sleep.
   ○ A special event like a birthday or going out to a restaurant.

3. Write down the story in your head at the moment of the trigger and the slip-up. What's going on in there? What's the story behind the story?

For example:

- *I've never been able to stick to something long term, so why bother trying? Failing in front of everyone so many times is demoralizing.*

- *I want to be able to go out with my friends and enjoy myself without worrying about calories or carbs.*

- *I'm lonely, but the idea of dating freaks me out. If I lose the weight, I'll have no excuse not to get out there.*

- *I'm not ready to give up my favorite foods forever. I'm worried I'll always feel deprived.*

4. Examine the thought. Is it true? How is it serving you? How does it keep you stuck?

5. What actions and results does that thought lead to?

For example:

- All or nothing thinking. "I already blew it so I might as well enjoy myself."

- Punishing yourself the next day, either in your thoughts or actions or both.

- Resolving to "be good" tomorrow, only to find yourself falling off again at dinner.

Sneaky Sabotagers

Weight loss is easier when you remove as many negative self-talk triggers as possible that cause self-sabotage. Negative self-talk is a powerful habit trigger.

Most of the time, knowing what to eat is not the key to weight loss.

The key to weight loss is in how we think about what we eat, what we tell ourselves about what we can and cannot eat or do, and what we make that mean about ourselves.

Watch out for statements that include:

- "I can't have..."
  - How many times have you looked at the "rules" of the diet du jour and realized that some special food you'd like to eat is on the "do not eat this" list? Whatever that food is, when you tell yourself "I CAN'T have it." you create a dichotomy in your brain.

    By telling yourself you can't have some type of food, you set yourself up for failure because you pit yourself against yourself. This is often what you feel on the weekend when you think "I just need a break!" You're tired from always having to obey the rules so the rebellious side of you wins out.

    Instead of telling yourself "I can't have X," try shifting your thoughts and words around.

    Words matter.

    The way you talk to yourself matters. Pay attention to the words you use in your head and out loud.

    Try saying "I choose to have X" or "I choose not to eat X."

    - Ex: *"I choose to eat birthday cake because I want to enjoy celebrating this special milestone with my daughter. I'll be present in the moment and really taste and not feel guilty about it. Because I'm present with it, I only need one piece to be satisfied."*

- Ex: *"I choose not to eat ice cream at the restaurant because I know that I won't feel so great in my body afterward and I choose getting a decent night's sleep versus reacting to what's right in front of me in the moment."*

- "I have to…"
  - This often comes out as *"I have to exercise"* or *"I have to watch what I'm eating."*

    It's the same principle as above. When you tell yourself you HAVE to do something, that puts the agency and control outside of yourself.

    We humans like to have a sense of control over our lives. By telling yourself, "I HAVE to X" you play the role of the victim in your own life.

    You get to write the story of your life. Do you want to play the role of the victim or the hero in your own life?

    Instead of saying "I have to X" try saying "I GET TO X."

    "I get to exercise because I like the way I feel afterwards. I get to go for a walk because I appreciate that my legs work, and I have the freedom of movement. I get to eat a salad at lunch because I like feeling lighter in my body."

    There are so many ways you can complete the sentence "I get to…." Fill in the rest of the sentence with something meaningful to you.

    When you attach a new meaning to your choices, they take on a whole new level of power and purpose.

- "I should..." or "they should…"
  - This sentence is really the same as the other two, only it adds a passive aggressive helping of guilt and shame as a side dish.

    Awesome.

    Whenever you catch yourself saying or thinking a "should" (shoulds are very sneaky!), try shifting that thought to one of the empowered ones from above.

    - Instead of *"I should go to the gym"* try *"I get to go to the gym"* or *"I choose not to go to the gym because my body is feeling sore from yesterday."*
    - Instead of *"I should set aside time to meal plan"* try *"I get to save myself the hassle of deciding later when I'm tired, so I choose to meal plan on Sunday at 10:30 before going to the grocery store."*
    - Instead of *"My mother shouldn't comment on what I eat."* try *"I choose to see my mother with compassion because she learned from her upbringing that looks are the only thing that matters."*

    Don't give yourself extra guilt and shame with the shoulds.

    Drop the shoulds and the victim mindset and take agency by focusing on what you can control and put yourself in the driver's seat of your choices, and thus, your life.
- "I'm worried about…."
  - Most of the things we worry about are outside our control and thus a waste of energy. Funnel that energy

into examining the things that you CAN control and then solve for those things. (Stay tuned for more on worry in a minute.)

- "What if I...."
  - ○ "What if's" are another version of worries. Only better because you can claim a little agency over the disempowering thought by adding a little action to the end of it.

    Whenever you catch yourself thinking "What if I....?" just add on what you'll do if that situation comes up.

    "What if X happens? Then I will ...."

Once you get to the real reasons why you're holding yourself back, then you can begin to redirect them.

TAKE IT FURTHER

For a fillable worksheet to identify and redirect sneaky sabotagers, go to https://confidentbody.coach/book/ and download your bonuses.

STEP 2: REDIRECT

How can you tell yourself a better story or ask yourself a better question to create better actions and results?

1. Challenge the thought.
Look for evidence that it might not be true.

For example:

- *I've never been able to stick to something long term, so why bother trying?*
  - You have figured out lots of other impressive things in your life. Whether it's how to raise a child, finish school, or complete a project at work, you've figured things out in the past. You've seen other people succeed at weight loss and you're just as smart and capable as they are. If they can figure it out, you can too.
- *I want to be able to go out with my friends and enjoy myself without worrying about calories or carbs.*
  - You can still go out. And you can plan ahead. Create a plan for yourself that includes the desires of (1) you now, (2) your future self who is in the moment wanting to let loose with your friends, and (3) future you the day after the night out? How can the three of you create a plan that is a compromise of all your desires?
- *I'm lonely, but the idea of dating freaks me out. If I lose the weight, I'll have no excuse not to get out there.*
  - What if your ideal partner is out there, just waiting for you to meet them? Fifty years from now, what will you regret more: feeling vulnerable by putting yourself out there and or never trying?
- *I'm not ready to give up my favorite foods forever. I'm worried I'll always feel deprived.*
  - Depriving yourself is not a sustainable plan. You can absolutely learn to have your favorite foods in moderation. If you hate your life as you're losing weight, you'll hate what it takes to keep the weight off.

2. Proactively choose a more empowering thought.

How can you take that old story in your head and look for an empowering alternative?

For example:

- *"I've never been able to stick to something long term, so why bother trying." becomes...*
  - ○ **I can figure this out. With every mistake, I'm learning and getting closer to my goal.**
- *"I want to be able to go out with my friends and enjoy myself without worrying about calories or carbs." becomes....*
  - ○ **I can always find ways to enjoy myself and keep promises to myself at the same time. I've always got my own back.**
- *"I'm lonely, but the idea of dating freaks me out. If I lose the weight, I'll have no excuse not to get out there." becomes....*
  - ○ **My future is worth fighting for.**
- *"I'm not ready to give up my favorite foods forever. I'm worried I'll always feel deprived." becomes.....*
  - ○ **"I can enjoy my favorite foods in a way that supports me."**

3. Use the old thought to your advantage.

Your brain has been practicing your old thought patterns for a long time. It is unrealistic to hope that the negative thoughts will just go away.

Having a negative thought is simply evidence that your brain is working properly. A negative thought is NOT evidence that you can't succeed.

We're gonna turn that negative thought pattern into a positive.

You have to deliberately practice new thinking. Just like you'd practice serving a tennis ball in order to get better at it, you need to proactively practice new thoughts.

Every time you have a negative thought about yourself or notice an old story coming up, you can use it as a trigger to choose a different thought.

It's **an invitation** to remind yourself, "We're not talking to ourselves that way anymore." And then program in and practice the more empowering thought.

YOUR REDIRECT ROUTINE

Here are some redirect examples for the four most common types of self-sabotaging thoughts:

Low self-esteem

Instead of telling yourself things that make you feel terrible, try asking a new question.

- If I believed I could succeed (even if I don't believe it right now), what would I do next?
- What would someone who has already been successful do?
- What advice would my wise, future self give me right now?

Fear of Failure

Instead of worrying about what might go wrong, how can you look at failure as a gift?

- What if each slip up is an invitation to learn about my triggers?
- What if each overeat is the roadmap to improvement?
- What if every time I fall off the wagon is actually a chance to practice the skill of getting right back on track?

Fear of Change

Rather than worrying about how things will change, try asking....

- What if I'm going to learn to like all kinds of foods, while not having to give up the ones I love? What if that could be possible?
- What could I imagine myself eating in six months that I'm not ready to try today?
- What's a way that I could lose weight in a way that my whole family loves what we eat? How can I make this work for all of us?
- How might I learn to go out to eat and enjoy myself on vacation and still feel healthy?

Fear of Success

Instead of thinking about how your body isn't what you want it to be, look for what IS right about you. Ask yourself....

- In what ways can I love and appreciate this body at any weight?

- What life is this body giving me?
- What is RIGHT about me (using all five of your senses, not just your eyes.)

It can be scary to let go of that weight when it was built to protect you to begin with. But when we build walls to keep out rejection or vulnerability, we also keep out all the good things – the good people, experiences, and feelings.

Ask yourself, *"At this time in my life, do I still need protection from the things I'm hiding from? Or can I learn to be resilient in my mind and take care of that person who felt like she needed a wall and tell her I got this now?"*

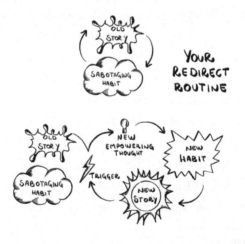

Remember the Reticular Activating System (RAS)?

Someone who believes they can lose weight looks for examples of how it's possible.

You can tell your brain what to filter for by proactively telling yourself a better story and by asking better questions. The brain is made to filter out and look for stuff that supports your story. So be very clear on what your story is.

Be careful where you point your brain's filter because whatever you're looking for, you'll find it.

STEP 3: PRACTICE

How long have you been carrying around those limiting beliefs? Probably years.

So how many times of repeating a new story would it take to rewrite the old story? Fortunately, it doesn't take years. But it does take proactive, conscious practice.

Overcoming self-sabotage may take a while, so don't be shocked or feel like you're doing it wrong. This takes practice. A lot of it.

Give yourself the grace to be terrible at this at first.

Each time you try to tell yourself a different story to create a different result (even when you fail many times over!) you're gradually telling your brain *"I'm interested in a new pattern. I'm willing to put in the time and effort to pull that old thought pattern up from my subconscious and purposefully create a new pattern."*

Even if it doesn't work right away (it probably won't work right away), practice telling yourself a new story.

Ask better questions.

Be patient. This takes time, repetition, and practice.

Be willing to fail time and again.

That's called LEARNING.

Common Crocodiles of Self Sabotage

Near St. Augustine Florida, there's a place called the Alligator Farm. The Alligator Farm is famous for some mighty large animals. Before he died, Gomek, the colossal saltwater crocodile was 17 ft 9 in. His successor, Maximo is a powerhouse at 15 ft 3 in. I don't know exactly how big Hagrid is, but I promise, he's impressive.

Just like these massive animals draw our attention and fascination because of their size, there are some common self-sabotaging thoughts that our brains can get stuck on because of how large they loom in our minds.

1) Falling Off the Wagon

Have you ever had a day where you started off great? You had a nice healthy breakfast. Things are going well through lunch. Then in the afternoon you have a few pretzels and realize that puts you over your calories for the day.

Suddenly you're thinking, "Ugh. I had three pretzel sticks instead of two, and that put me twenty-three calories over my budget. The heck with it. I really wanted potato chips anyway. And while I'm at it (since I've already blown it), I might as well have three cupcakes, a half a box of crackers, and three slices of pizza."

This all or nothing thinking is so common, psychologists have even named it the "what-the-hell-effect".[22] When you've made a "bad" choice and feel guilty about it, you give up on trying to eat well because, "What the hell. The day is already ruined."

---

22 https://www.psychologytoday.com/us/blog/pressure-proof/201701/how-the-what-the-hell-effect-impacts-your-willpower

Basically, we tell ourselves, *"I fell off the wagon. Now I have to start over from scratch."*

Then you vow to start "fresh" the next morning... or Monday... or next week...or after the holidays, etc.

All or nothing thinking is one of the BIGGEST challenges of dieting.

It's like if you were trying to teach your seven-year-old how to ride a bike. But your adorable little daughter tells you, *"Okay Mommy! I'm ready to learn how to ride a bike. However, I don't want to fall. Not once. And actually, I need to be able to ride blindfolded and have this feel easy by my second try. Okay? Great, let's go."*

We expect ourselves to be perfect with lots of changes all at once.

I don't know about you, but that's definitely NOT how my kids learned to ride bikes. (In fact, we lovingly called our son "Pepperoni Pizza Face" for a while since he managed to scrape up his face on the sidewalk a few times.)

Listen. Weight loss includes screws-ups.

Expect it. Plan for it. Accept yourself for it.

What do you think is the main difference between people who are successful at weight loss and those who are not?

- It's not how well they followed their plan.
- It's not how many mistakes or slip-ups they had.

The main difference is the people who are successful simply KEPT GOING.

That's it.

Just keep going. Keep going and your goals are inevitable.

Being able to not quit is **The Skill** of weight loss.

You don't drown by falling in the water.
You drown from staying there.
~Steve Sims

Beating yourself up every time you make a mistake eventually leads to quitting. Instead of trying to be perfect, let's acknowledge two important things:

1. You are the product of the things you do every day, not the things you do every once in a while. If you occasionally do something outside of your norm (like eat a plate full of cookies, skip a workout, etc.), that one moment won't have a lasting impact on your health.

2. A splurge will only affect your progress when you keep indulging. Step number one is always forgive yourself. Then only focus on your NEXT choice. Just focusing on the next choice feels less overwhelming than recommitting to your "diet" forever.

3. Don't diet. Diets perpetuate all or nothing thinking because of all the rules it imposes on you. When you subscribe to all or nothing thinking, you're susceptible to falling off the wagon. Instead of the Diet Mentality, give the Next Best Decision mentality a try.

You're never more than your next best choice away from being right back on track. Rather than going into full on "screw it" mode, just look for the next best decision.

Maybe your next best decision is to stop with one Dorito left in the bag. Maybe the next best decision is to wake up tomorrow and make a positive choice, rather than say "Well I messed up on Friday night so I might as well eat what I want until Monday."

The next best decision can always be to tell yourself that your past does not define your future. Whether it was the last twenty years or the last twenty minutes, you always have a new opportunity in front of you to choose yourself. And the next best decision can always include loving yourself, no matter how imperfect you are.

You don't need to wait till Monday. What's the next best choice you can make in the next ten minutes?

When I was in my phase of constantly seeking the "after picture", I found that I'd do well for three to five weeks or so, but then something would come along and wreck my progress.

A trip to visit family, someone got sick, a holiday. Always something. It was really frustrating to feel like I was gaining momentum, only to have it derailed by some random thing.

After a while, I began to notice a pattern.

These progress-upsetting events always seemed to come along after about threeish weeks of "being good." I began to wonder if maybe I was thinking about things backwards. I was thinking that the events were abnormal, unusual disruptions to my routine.

But because they were so predictable, maybe they weren't so abnormal after all. I mean, life can be predictably unpredictable. That's life!!

It's understandable to have slip-ups when you're not feeling well or unexpected life events get in the way. It can be frustrating to feel like you're on track and have a good week or two and then something like a trip or an illness comes along and wrecks all your progress.

It's tempting to think that the thing that comes along is out of the ordinary.

But another way to look at it is that life is full of periodic events that disrupt our routines.

Whether it's a stressful week at work or family comes to town or the dog pooped on the floor.

It can be helpful to think of those disruptive moments as a very normal and predictable part of life.

If these events are predictable, then you can plan for them. What if you assumed that life and all its interruptions are normal? Life's default mode (without inputting extra effort) is to be less conscious of your food, exercise, sleep, health, etc.

It's like pedaling a bicycle. If you keep pedaling, the bike will keep going. But the natural default is for the bike to slow down and eventually stop and fall over if you don't pedal.

So there's no reason to be upset with yourself for getting slowed down by life's natural default! It's normal!!

You can be aware that healthy habits simply take consistent pedaling. You don't have to go very fast to keep the bike going, but it does take a little pedaling to avoid falling back into default.

If you were to make the assumption that something will eventually come along and disrupt your routine, how can you look at it as something that is expected? Then you can make a plan for how you'll keep pedaling your bicycle just a little bit to help you get right back on track.

Just like a kid learning to ride a bike, you can figure out how to fail, make mistakes, slip up, and keep going.

The only difference between someone who loses weight and someone who doesn't is that in the moment that they overeat or make a mistake, one of them keeps going, and the other one gives up on themselves.

The person who succeeds is able to be present and have a better conversation with themselves.

If you hang on to the Diet Mentality and the idea that you have to be perfect, then you fail. The magic lies in the willingness to keep going until you figure it out. How can you learn to become the person who is figuring it out a little bit at a time?

Your secret weapon against all or nothing thinking is self-compassion.[23] Self-compassion does not mean you're making excuses for yourself, nor does it led to more "cheat days."

Even though it is easy to assume that you need to be hard on yourself to get anything done, we already know that self-criticism is strongly associated with LESS self-control and motivation.[24] In other words, beating yourself up means you're LESS likely to change your ways.

It's a lose-lose.

On the other hand, being kind to yourself and offering yourself self-compassion gives you a greater sense of agency, self-efficacy, and motivation. (That's fancy talk for *"I can DO IT!"* or at least, *"I think I can figure this out. I'll try again."*)

---

23 Self Compassion by Kristin Neff
24 The Willpower Instinct by Kelly McGonigal

We ALL fall off the wagon. The key to getting back "on the wagon" is forgiveness and self-compassion, not guilt, shame, and harsh criticism.

Speaking of falling off the wagon...did you know that the phrase "falling off the wagon" comes from the 1890s during the height of the temperance movement when folks advocated for complete abstinence from alcohol as part of the anti-saloon league?[25]

The "water wagon" was actually used for sanitation purposes to hose down dusty streets. Let's just say this water was not purified Aqua Fina drinking water. So if you were "on the wagon," that meant you were so committed to not drinking alcohol that you'd rather drink the gross water from the sanitation cart than drink alcohol. Obviously, it's taken on other meanings since then and now includes the idea of falling "off" your diet.

But here's the problem with that notion: It implies that you're just riding merrily along and "*Oops! We hit a bump and fell off.*" The phrase implies that something happened TO you. That's secretly self-sabotage, because you're putting the power somewhere else outside of you. "*It's not MY fault I fell off the wagon. We hit a bump!*" It's like you're at the mercy of your environment.

You always have a choice. Even if that choice to act on your desires is buried in your subconscious habits, it's still a choice to respond and act on an urge. If it's a choice, then it's not just happening TO you. You have control.

When you DO cave and act on the desire (you will, and that's okay) it's tempting to say, "*I just fell off the wagon. It's no big deal.*

25 https://www.mentalfloss.com/article/640247/fall-off-the-wagon-phrase-origin

I'll just get back on tomorrow." While that's better than berating yourself, take a second to stop. Slow down and reflect!

Never let a slip-up go to waste. Your subconscious mind wants you to blow it off and not be aware of what might have led up to that event. The longer you leave it in your unconscious mind, the more it's gonna feel like it's out of your voluntary control.

Unravel the thread. Use your prefrontal cortex to pay attention and examine everything that went on leading up to "falling off the wagon." Be like a scientist! Learn from your experiments.

"We can do hard things."
~Glennon Doyle

Often, falling off the wagon is not really the problem. It's the challenge of getting "back on the wagon" that trips us up.

Have you ever seen a toddler learning to walk?

They may take a few steps and then fall on their rear end. It's normal! It's part of the process. The next time, they take a few more steps and still fall down. They get back up and try again.

What if a baby had the same attitude that we take toward weight loss? *"Why can't I get this right?!?"* They'd never learn to walk because they would give up after the first stumble!

There is nothing wrong with you when you have a slip-up or fall off the wagon. It's normal! Falling down and taking backward steps is an expected part of the learning process. The real skill is getting back up again. Learn the skill of getting back up and you never need to fear falling off the wagon again.

2) Food Labeling

Have you ever heard yourself say "*I was bad this weekend.*"?

What the heck does that even mean? Did you rob a bank? Steal candy from babies? Sing Brittney Spears songs at a karaoke bar???

Let's just start with the words themselves:

"Good"

"Bad"

There's a lot of baggage associated with those words. When you label a food (or yourself when you eat that food) as "good" or "bad," you're associating a sense of morality to that food.

Along with that comes guilt and shame.

If we take it at its most basic level, food, no matter what kind, is a collection of energy that impacts our body in different ways. Whether you're looking at a donut or an apple, the body looks at both of them as forms of energy.

If we take it one step further, one is more nourishing to the body than the other based on the collection of nutrients in it.

But they're still both energy. Not good or bad. Just nourishing or less nourishing.

Then our brains get in the mix when we make the level of nourishment MEAN something about the food or about ourselves when we eat it.

We attach a sense of morality to food that is over and above whether or not it is nourishing to the body.

What would it be like to let go of the shame and guilt associated with food and try and look at it from the point of view of "more nourishing" or "less nourishing"?

Food is <u>NOT</u> just fuel. Food can be a source of community, love, safety, shared experiences.

That's why no food is "bad."

Part of living a full life is enjoying the foods you love. But the idea is to eat them when you're actually hungry and truly enjoy them, versus eating in secret or as comfort and not ever really tasting them. Most of us overeat because we're trying to solve our feelings with food.

Give yourself the respect to know that your feelings are important and worth paying attention to, rather than stuffing them away with food.

3) I Don't Want to Let Food Go To Waste

Have you ever finished the box of crackers or the package of cookies, just to get it out of the house?

Why eat it instead of just throwing it away?

A lot of us have internal scripts that we learned when we were young about "clean your plate" or "don't let food go to waste."

Whether it's from messages we got from our parents or financial insecurity, there can be all kinds of reasons why we think it's wrong to throw food away.

Whatever the reason, it can be hard to "let food go to waste."

Imagine you had guests come visit and after they leave, there's some leftover food in the pantry that is less-than-healthy. Normally it wouldn't be there, but you had it because the guests were visiting.

It can be tempting to tell yourself *"I'll just eat this to get rid of it and finish it off. I don't want to waste it by throwing it away."* (I've totally done this.) So the choice is either (a) eat it or (b) throw it away.

Here's the thing:

When you decide to eat it instead of throwing it away, you're using your body as the garbage can.

The food is a sunk cost. The money is already spent, no matter if you put it in your mouth or the garbage. Putting it in your body to get your money's worth doesn't affect your wallet, nor does it help your body.

Eating it doesn't mean that you got more for your money. It just means you put extra calories in your body.

The first time I heard this idea it really blew me away.

But why do we have so much trouble with the thought distortion around not wanting to waste food? How are we all so disconnected from what it means to have "enough" and not feel compelled to have more, just because it's there?

Ever heard of the Clean Plate Club? Maybe you heard grandpa proudly announce after Sunday dinner, *"I'm a member of the Clean Plate Club! How about you? You gonna finish that pork chop?"*

It turns out the Clean Plate Club really existed. As WWI was winding down, Woodrow Wilson created the US Food Administration to help ration food and make sure that the limited post-war supplies did not go to waste.

Future president Herbert Hoover was tasked with leading the organization, and he created an advertising campaign promoting the idea to "clean your plate" to school age children. They even had kids sign clean plate pledges. "Food will win the war. Don't waste it."[26] The campaign was used again during the depression and WWII.

It's crazy how that messaging got passed down to many of us today, even though we grew up in an environment where food was plentiful instead of scarce.

Why is your brain clinging to the idea that wasting is so wrong? Is your brain still holding on to a message that got passed to you through your parents from their parents before them and maybe even their parents before that when circumstances were very different from what they are today?

Never wasting food is an easy rule to live by. It feels like a smart idea. However, it disconnects you from your body and from knowing how much is "enough."

Finishing your plate, or the bag of chips, or the bottle of wine leaves those old patterns and stories in your subconscious where it's hard to do anything about them.

Examining those thought patterns takes work.

Your goals are on the other side of awareness.

4) Worry

"What if I gain it all back?"

"What if I fail….again?"

Ah, my ol' pal Worry.

Worry is tomorrow's fear showing up today.

Worry is our subconscious mind's way of searching for a guarantee. It's wanting a promise that the end result will be worth all the hard work.

---

26 Food Conservation during WWI: "Food Will Win the War" https://www.gilderlehrman.org/news/food-conservation-during-wwi-food-will-win-war

If you've ever worried whether or not you can keep the weight off or if you'll backslide again, the fear in the back of your mind is completely normal and it's okay that it's there.

When we push fear away or try to ignore it, it comes in the back door and sabotages our efforts. Instead of pushing fear away, allow it to be there.

Liz Gilbert, author of *Eat, Pray, Love*, talks about fear and anxiety in a way that really resonates for me.

"Fear is allowed to have a voice, but not a vote. Me, courage, and fear – we're all going on an adventure together. Fear is allowed a seat, but under no circumstances is it allowed to drive."
~Liz Gilbert

It is important to address these fears and look at them in the light of day. If you've trained your brain to repeat the pattern of worry or angst, then even if you do lose weight, your brain will still be stuck in the old pattern, just a new refrain.

It'll worry about whether you can keep the weight off or worry how long it will last. Your brain will look for the smallest of mistakes and blow them out of proportion.

This is why it is SO important to address your mindset when you're embarking on a lifestyle change. Who wants to get their goal and then still feel miserable when they get there?

By worrying about the future, you are training yourself to not be happy with the present.

Let's say you've lost ten pounds, but you have more you want to lose.

I bet if I asked you several months ago, "How happy would you be if you lost ten pounds?" You'd say "Very happy!"

And yet here you are, having lost the ten pounds, and worry for tomorrow is stealing your happiness today.

How can you create a narrative that allows for fear to be there and allows courage and self-compassion to be just a little bit bigger, stronger, and louder than that fear? When you do that, you begin to trust yourself and allow yourself to feel great about how far you've come.

When those thoughts come up, it's not a problem. It's a signal. It's an invitation to proactively choose a thought that is more constructive and helpful for you.

Brains need supervision and direction. Your brain is a tool, and it does what it's told. If you don't deliberately tell it what to do, it'll do what it's always done and create what it's always created. Recognizing that your brain needs supervision and direction on a daily basis is really important.

Every time you feel the thought "I can't succeed" or "I am afraid that I will fail again" try telling yourself "I have no idea what I am capable of."

It doesn't work until it actually works.

Have a better conversation with yourself. You won't know if the process works until you do it. If you've got to be scared while you do it, then be scared. That's okay! But having a better conversation with yourself must be the place to start, because I guarantee you that keeping those old self-loathing thoughts will lead you down the same path you've always been.

Expecting to be fearless is perfectionist thinking. Every time you try something new there is going to be fear or worry there because it's new. You've never tried it before.

The fear is there, and it gets a voice. But it doesn't get a vote.

5) Comparison

> *"Comparison is the thief of joy."*
> *~Teddy Roosevelt*

Preach, Teddy!

While ole Teddy may have been absolutely right that comparison feels like poop, he didn't take into account that it's kinda wired into our DNA to compare ourselves to others.

Honestly, until I learned how our human brains naturally compare ourselves to others, that quote has always made me feel a little guilty. As usual, it all goes back to prehistoric times. In the old days, you needed to compare yourself to others to make sure you were fitting in with the tribe. If you didn't fit in and were left behind, that literally meant death.

So it's not my fault that I compare myself to others! Ha ha, in your face Teddy Roosevelt!

However, it still feels lousy when I compare myself to others and find myself falling short. That's because, in those moments, I'm letting comparison turn my thoughts toward envy. I've seen this show up in myself and with my clients in two ways.

1) Disdain for someone who has what you want.
   Remember when I said that we lived in Guam for a military assignment? If you're not familiar with Guam, it's

a teeny, tiny island amid a vast ocean. It's wonderful as long as you're good with constantly being sweaty, sandy, or your hair is messed up by the wind. Given those factors, I pretty much wore a baseball hat and workout clothes every day for an entire year.

Each day when I'd go to pick my kids up at school, there was this mom there who always looked put together. Here she was looking like she had showered (gasp!), put on makeup, and even brushed her hair. Meanwhile I looked like a hot, sweaty mess. So my subconscious mind decided that I hated her instantly. (Did I mention she also had the perfect body?)

Here's the problem with that:

Your brain will never let you become something you disdain. So my brain got the message that *"Being showered, put together, and looking cute for pre-school pick up is bad."*

Therefore, my brain subconsciously implemented the operating program titled: *"We will avoid looking cute at all costs."*

Is that really what I wanted to tell my brain to think about? Of course not. But that's the crazy thing that happens when we try and protect ourselves from comparison by disdaining someone or something that makes us feel less than.

It turns out that "Cute Mom" was actually super nice. Figures.

Who is someone you've assumed is a "skinny b****" or thought "it's easy for her" because she looks the way you'd like to? Bring those thoughts up to the surface where you can see them.

Your brain will literally prevent you from becoming something you disdain. So instead, how can you look at this person as someone you can relate to? What do you like about them? How can you humanize them so that whatever they've achieved seems more attainable to your subconscious mind rather than *"Nope. Never gonna happen."*

2) Feeling jealous of someone else's progress.

Being part of a weight loss group can be amazing. It helps to have the support of others who "get it" and are going through the same things as you.

However, I've often had clients that are in group coaching come to me and say, *"Everyone in my group is having more success than I am. I should be losing weight faster. I feel like I am doing it wrong. I'm so demoralized."*

Listen, it is human nature to compare ourselves to others. However, using other people's successes as evidence of why you can't do it is a sure path to failure. That's bound to make you feel bad and want to quit.

Here are a few strategies to help you with comparison:

1) Perspective

When our daughter was in sixth grade, about ¾ of the way through the first semester, she decided that she wanted to try playing trumpet in the band. So we jumped through the hoops to get her transferred into band class, rented her a trumpet, and said, *"Follow your dreams, Young Adventurer!"*

However, when she got into band, she soon felt waaaaay behind the other kids because she'd never picked up a trumpet before in her life and these kids already had a semester (or more) of practice under their belt.

When you compare yourself to others, you're often comparing your beginning to someone else's middle.

Of course you're not as far along as they are! They've been working at this for longer or they have different environmental factors going on.

There are so many things that make their story different from yours. Comparing yourself to them is like saying apple trees are lame because they don't grow as tall as pine trees. Whaaa? That doesn't make any sense.

Love yourself enough to give your dream time and space to grow, mature, evolve, and succeed.

2) Eyes on your own paper.

My freshman year in college I was taking an intro calculus class. As you might imagine, a calculator was extremely helpful. Being the mega nerd that I am, I sat in the front row of my eight a.m. class to make sure I didn't fall asleep during lecture.

One day we were having a quiz and I had forgotten to get my calculator out of my backpack before the quiz began. As I bent over to grab it, (I swear I did not do this on purpose) my gaze brushed past the paper on my neighbor's table. "Oh crap!" I thought. "I SO did not mean to do that. Now it looks like I cheated when I was just not paying attention when I bent down to get my stupid calculator."

Fortunately, nothing happened. I did not see anything from their page and the teacher did not bust me for roving eyes.

The moral of the story is nothing good comes from looking over someone else's shoulder. When you do that you either:

a) Question yourself. *"How is she so much further along than I am? I'm not losing weight fast enough."*

b) Or you feel juuuust a little bit, kinda sorta superior to them. And that's not the most jolly of feelings either.

Focus on YOUR journey. Someone else's progress (or lack thereof) just isn't relevant to what you're doing.

3) Flip it to inspiration.

What if comparison is like looking through binoculars backward and it makes your goal seem soooo much farther away? Instead, flip those suckers around and look at your situation in a way that makes your goal seem closer.

Use someone else's progress as INSPIRATION.

What if you consciously used someone else's success as a way to inspire you? What if their progress is evidence of what's possible?

How much better does this thought feel? *"If they can do it, then maybe I can too!"*

Choose thoughts that set you up for success, not failure.

> *"You can't be half envious and half grateful."*
> ~Dan Sullivan

Comparing yourself to others can be useful if you use it as a source of insight and possibility rather than using it as a weapon against yourself. Envy is demoralizing and gives you a sense of scarcity in the world where someone else's gain is a loss for you. When you find envy creeping in, turn toward gratitude.

Be grateful for what that person's accomplishment means for what is possible for you. Be grateful for the ideas that their success can give you to serve you on your path. Someone who is further along the path can be inspiring to you if you cultivate gratitude.

There's no competition on the field of gratitude because everyone wins. There's enough for everyone to win and step into their full self when you use that feeling of envy as an opportunity for gratitude.

There is only ONE of you.

When there is only one of something, it cannot be compared. You don't have to feel like you need to compare yourself to others because you are literally incomparable.

You are a perfect representation of the Divine.

6) Vanity

When I met Susan, she was already an accomplished athlete. She had participated in triathlons and enjoyed the idea of competing.

However, life had thrown her a few curveballs and she'd put on about ten pounds from what she felt like was her ideal weight.

When I asked her about her goals, she hesitated. *"I don't know,"* she said. *"I mean, I know I'm still in relatively good shape. And I should feel grateful for that."*

Whenever I hear a "should," it makes me curious. So I said, *"Tell me more about that."*

"Well, it feels kinda vain to want to get lean so I can be competitive again when I already have a really healthy body."

Ah! Now we were getting somewhere. As we dug deeper, we uncovered an old script in Susan's mind that said, *"Wanting to look good is vain. And vanity is bad."* She realized that she felt selfish if she spent time in pursuit of good looks and it made her feel like she was being superficial.

Can you imagine how these thoughts might hold Susan back from feeling good about herself? Over time, her self-judgment made it hard to prioritize taking time for herself to look and feel better.

We get very mixed messages from society. It is important to look good. Looking good is a type of currency. And yet if we *think* we look good or want to look sexy then we're egotistical. You have to look good while not actually thinking you look good. It's a no-win situation!

It's understandable to feel a little conflicted about that.

"Most have shame triggers around being perceived as self-indulgent or self-focused. We don't want our authenticity to be perceived as selfish or narcissistic."
~Brene Brown

Here are some questions to consider:

Is it selfish to feel confident, at ease in your body, and proud of yourself?

- What would you tell a young woman (maybe your daughter or a niece?) if she wanted to feel confident and proud of herself? Would you tell her that she is selfish?

- How does feeling confident in your body free you up to live authentically and bring your best self into this world?

Wanting to look and feel good is not egotistical. It's wanting to show up in the world as your best self. There's nothing wrong with that!!

Bringing your FULL self to the world and offering your gifts with confidence is one of the most valuable things you can do in this life.

If you've ever felt like Susan and worried that wanting to look good makes you selfish, how might you examine the thoughts about superficiality and selfishness as possibly someone else's scripts that you learned from somewhere else? Maybe they're not your truth.

You can choose your own truth.

What would you LIKE to believe about what it means to care for your body and care about your appearance?

7) Permission

Sarah leaned in close and said, *"My biggest struggle is permission. Just feeling like it's okay to take time to care for myself can be a big hurdle sometimes."*

Sarah is the mom of two girls, wife to a husband that works 72 hours a week to support their family, and oh by the way, she also owns her own business. Needless to say, Sarah is a busy gal.

Like so many of us, Sarah is a doer. A helper. She is the one who makes sure that everyone is taken care of. If a ball drops, she's on it. If a kid is sick, she's nursing them back to health.

On top of that, she knows all sorts of science about the body and how food impacts her cells and hormones. But when it comes to taking action, all that knowledge ain't got nothin' in the face of the demands and stressors of life.

When there is always someone in need or something that needs to get done, how can Sarah decide to say, "No. I'm not helping you or fixing this right now because I am taking care of me."?

How do we give ourselves permission to put ourselves first? Or even permission to allow ourselves to feel good with self-care (massage anyone?)

When Sarah and I talked through this, she said, *"I feel like I don't deserve it. Like why should I be better than or higher than my family in terms of my priorities?"*

Sarah also has a deep faith in God and has a servant's heart. So I asked her, *"How would God answer that question about 'why you should be higher than your family' in terms of priorities?"*

That made her pause.

"I've never thought of it that way before."

(Long pause.)

"Wow. I think He would say that I am His beloved child just as much as anyone in my family. Why should I deserve any less than any of them?"

(Another long pause.)

"Holy cow. I could even say that God would tell me that I am His divine instrument. I am beautifully and wonderfully made. Handcrafted by Him. The Bible even says that our bodies are a temple of the Holy Spirit. Who am I to say that God is wrong?"

What a powerful moment.

All the knowledge, all the science, all the guilt and shame that Sarah had accumulated over the years did not have the power to overcome her story that she needed to put everyone else first.

It was her commitment to God that helped her see that she not only has permission to say no to other things in favor of caring for herself, she is commanded to do so by her faith.

With God, all things are possible. And sometimes we need to realize that loving and caring for ourselves is an act of love, care, and obedience to God as well.

"Do you not know that your bodies are temples of the Holy Spirit,
who is in you, whom you have received from God?"
~1 Corinthians 6:19

Sometimes the hardest part is to receive.

You know that feeling when you give your child or someone you love a gift? It's so fun to watch as he or she opens their present. It feels so good to see them love it and be really excited about it!

What if God is like that with us?

When we don't give ourselves permission to receive, we're like a kid who gets a gift and says "Oh. Uh, thanks. But I don't really need this. And I need to be doing my homework." What a downer.

What if everything in your life (including your body) is like a present from God on Christmas morning and He just can't wait to see your eyes light up and feel your joy in reveling in the awesomeness of His gift? How does God feel when He gives you a gift and you're like "Oh I don't deserve this."

Receiving is SUPPOSED to feel good!

What if each day is an opportunity to be that kid who is just so excited about their gifts and make God feel really awesome at the same time?

> *"...but put your hope in God, who richly provides us*
> *with everything for our enjoyment."*
> *1 Timothy 6:17*

"Okay, but how? I've already got too much on my plate. Where and when am I going to find the time to take care of me?"

I get it. Life is busy. There always seems to be something "extra" going on that derails any tiny bit of progress you might have had going. Someone is sick, the sink is leaking, and you're trying to sell your house...it can get overwhelming.

And yet we never ask for help.

We just say, "I'm so stressed."

I don't know about you, but I am much more comfortable offering help than asking for help. Why is that?

I mean, it feels good to help. That makes sense.

But maybe, it feels just a tiny bit vulnerable to ask for help and I might have to give away a little of my Scarlett O'Hara drama of, *"I did SO much today! Woe is me!"*

Yeah, my husband has been very clear on just how humorous he finds that act of martyrdom. (I'm trying to get better about it.)

If you love to help others, how do you think others feel when they get to help you?

Usually, they feel pretty darn awesome! It is part of our human nature to want to help. Helping intrinsically makes us feel good.

By allowing someone to help, you are giving them the gift of feeling good, feeling useful, feeling needed. Everyone wants to feel needed.

How can you shift your thoughts away from *"I am a burden to others if I ask for help"* and toward *"By asking for help, I am giving someone an opportunity to feel amazing."*?

By asking for help, we ask others to share their gifts with us and give them a chance to be in service. That can be a beautiful thing.

Not only that, but how do you show up when you feel like you're doing everything, you're exhausted all the time, and taking everything on your shoulders? How do your loved ones want you to show up for them? Tired and resentful or refreshed and present?

What would happen if you took time for yourself? Who would you be when you show up for others after taking time to care for yourself?

- It doesn't serve you or your loved ones to think of taking time for yourself as taking away from them.
- It doesn't serve you or them to tell yourself that there is something more valuable that you *should* be doing instead of taking care of you.

What if by putting yourself first, you are being better to those you love?

What if asking for help and allowing yourself to be helped so that you can take care of yourself is the best gift you can give them?

You charge your phone every night because you know that if you don't, the battery will run out and render it useless. Shouldn't you get the chance to recharge too?

We've all heard the commandment to *"Love your neighbor as yourself."* Most of my life I viewed that from the perspective of *"Be nice to other people."*

But as I've grown older, it seems like a lot of people (women especially) are able to be nice to others, but NOT to themselves.

What if the commandment is telling you to *"Love yourself in the same way that you love others"*?

You have something special that only YOU can bring to the world. By taking care of yourself, you are giving yourself permission to be all of YOU and bring your unique light to shine on others in your special way.

CHAPTER 9
HOW TO STOP EATING YOUR FEELINGS

Fairy Godmother:
STOP THE CAR!
(menacing voice) *Harold, you have forced me to do something I reeeeally don't want to do.*

King:
What...Wait...Where are we?

Fast Food Clerk:
Well, hi there! Welcome to Medieval Friar. May I take your order?

Fairy Godmother:
My diet is ruined! I hope you're happy.[27]

Chocolate Therapy

In 2013 my husband Steve was deployed to Bahrain. Usually, he would deploy on a ship and the family members back home would create a community to support each other.

---

27 Shrek 2, 2004 Dreamworks Studios

This was not like that.

He was deployed solo to a small staff on the other side of the world. So back home, there were no other families in the same situation.

We were on our own.

He'd been gone for about two months when Halloween rolled around. The kids looked adorable in their costumes. Our son was a ninja. Our daughter was dressed as Thomas the Train.

We walked the neighborhood, and they filled their jack-o-lantern buckets with all sorts of goodies. As I took pictures, all I could think was "Steve is missing this."

And I was missing him.

Later that night, after giving them a chance to enjoy some of their candy, I put the kids to bed.

I was tired too, but I just couldn't face going to bed alone.

So I stayed up.

I watched mindless TV way past when I'd normally go to bed.

The kids' candy was just there.

Staring at me.

So I ate chocolate.

Lots and lots of chocolate.

Grief Bacon

Why do we eat our feelings?

It's human nature to seek pleasure and avoid pain. Our neural systems are wired that way to help keep us alive. When we get stressed, our brains want relief from those painful feelings.

Watching Netflix feels better than feeling stressed, or sad. Eating mindlessly feels better than feeling bored.

Food is a quick and reliable source of dopamine, which feels good. So when you're feeling a negative emotion the brain can send up a thought that says "I know what will help! FOOD!"

<u>**Fun fact:**</u>

The German language actually has a word for this. It's called *kummerspeck,* which loosely translates to "*the weight we gain when feeling emotionally sad.*" The literal English translation is "*grief bacon.*"

I think that pretty much sums it up perfectly.

However, the way that food is designed these days, it over-stimulates the dopamine receptor sites. Overtime, the brain down-regulates the receptor sites (almost like developing a tolerance for alcohol) and thus when you have a little of the treat, the brain says "gimme more".

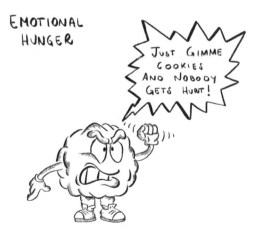

Emotional hunger is just as real as physical hunger, but the root cause is different. Therefore, trying to satisfy emotional hunger with food doesn't actually solve the issue.

How can you tell if you're feeling physically hungry or emotionally hungry?

Physical hunger is based in the body, comes on gradually, and is open to all foods. Eating an apple would help you feel satisfied.

Emotional hunger tends to be for a specific kind of food, like a craving. It comes up quickly. It tends to be paired with upsetting emotions. Feels urgent. It feels impatient and often having "just one" of the food doesn't quite satisfy the feeling. Emotional hunger often comes associated with feeling of guilt later.

Have you ever finished an apple and thought "I could eat six more of those"? I haven't. But I certainly have that feeling about Hersey's Kisses.

Emotional hunger is when you find yourself staring at the pantry thinking, "What do I want to eat?" without really remembering the conscious act of getting there.

You're more likely to fall prey to emotional hunger later in the day because your willpower tank is running on fumes and it's harder to make decisions.

Solving emotional hunger with food just covers up the problem and pretends it's not there. Since the root cause of emotional hunger is based in an emotional need rather than a physical one, the solution needs to address your feelings, not your food.

Ask yourself "Why am I eating?"

When you go to reach for food, try and notice why you're eating. Then make a proactive choice on whether or not you still choose to eat whatever the food is.

Just getting a feel for the various reasons WHY you might be tempted to eat can help you gain a lot of awareness into the difference between emotional hunger and physical hunger.

Sometimes we invalidate our feelings or diminish the stress we feel because, "Well, someone else has it worse" or "I shouldn't complain" etc.

No one wins the "Most Stressed" award.

The stress you feel is real. It doesn't matter if someone else might have a more stressful job or if your circumstances are really pretty great in general.

You're still feeling stress and ignoring it is like pretending the drain isn't getting clogged up. Over time, that gook in the drain (or stress in the body) accumulates unless you address it.

Thoughts are the language of the mind.

Emotions are the language of the body.

They both matter.

Emotions are just like anyone else. They want to be validated and heard. If you ignore them, they'll keep knocking on your door until you address them.

So give yourself some credit and validate your feelings!

Willpower and White Bears

Food and drink are glamorized in our society. It's everywhere. It can be birthday cake or Doritos or a glass of cabernet. Ads and media portray it as "You'll be happier if you have some."

Whether it's sugar or chips or alcohol, there is the unspoken assumption that you should be able to consume a proven addictive substance "without having a problem". So there's a stigma around not feeling one hundred percent in control of the craving.

And yet so many of us live in quiet torment thinking, "There's something wrong with me" because there is this competing desire between wanting it and wanting to NOT want it.

You start the day thinking "I will be good today. I'm definitely NOT having sugar today." And then later, the craving sneaks in. You second guess yourself.

Afternoon-Self negotiates with Morning-Self.

By 4:43 p,m., Morning-Self is exhausted. She's worn out from the demands of the day and Afternoon-Self has a different agenda. Whether it's sugar cookies or chardonnay, it's like you want it against your own will.

Ironically, battling against the desire actually INCREASES the desire. When you tell yourself you "can't" have chips or ice cream or whatever, that creates a dichotomy in yourself between the rebel who wants it and the tyrant who says "NO!" No matter who is winning in the moment, part of you is losing.

In her book titled *The Willpower Instinct* Kelly McGonigal, PhD explains how telling ourselves we "can't" have something actually makes us think about it MORE.

In an experiment conducted by Harvard psychologist Daniel Wegner, study participants were asked to NOT think about a white bear. Anything else was fair game. Just not a white bear.

As you may have guessed, the students failed miserably at trying NOT to think about white bears.[28]

Wegner coined the phrase *ironic rebound* to describe when we try not to think of something, we end up thinking about it even more.

Here's what's happening in the brain:

When you try not to think about something (like ice cream) you send a message to the subconscious mind to look out for any thoughts of ice cream. What this does is keeps the thought of ice cream front and center because the subconscious mind is always on alert for it.

Trying to suppress thoughts of ice cream (or chips or wine or whatever) is a double blow to your self-control.

1) It constantly brings the thought of the forbidden thing to mind. That means that you're not making one decision not to have the ice cream. Instead, you're forcing yourself to decide over and over again whether or not to have the ice cream.

2) This leads to decision fatigue. Making decisions (about anything-much less deciding to avoid ice cream) drains willpower. So by telling yourself NOT to think about ice cream, you're draining your willpower. Meaning before long, you've got nothing left in your willpower tank to make a proactive choice and you inevitably end up plunging into the freezer for the tub of ice cream.

3) In addition, we often don't understand the difference between battling against the desire and learning the tools to

---

28 The Willpower Instinct by Kelly McGonigal

address it. That struggle creates anxiety, and that anxiety creates more reason to want to eat or drink.

We unwittingly create a self-perpetuating cycle. Have a thought about sugar ⇒ struggle ⇒ creates anxiety ⇒ give in (or want more) to solve the anxiety ⇒ strengthen the neural pathway for turning to sugar.

Crazy, right?

Oddly enough, the solution to the dilemma is to allow yourself to think about whatever it is. Make it okay for thoughts about the food you're craving to come and go in your mind.

Wait, what?

That sounds terrible!

Actually, if you're willing to get curious, the key to your freedom lies on the other side of a little discomfort.

Doggie Drool and Cravings

Back in the day when Pavlov was experimenting on his dogs, he noticed that the dogs learned to expect food when the bell rang. He could tell they were expecting food because they were salivating. Over time, the dogs mentally connected the bell with food. So the bell triggered their DESIRE for food, as evidenced by the salivating.

The same thing happens in our brain. There is an automatic response. Trigger leads to desire.

- Trigger: It's 4:37 p.m. on a Friday
  - Desire: I want a glass of wine.
- Trigger: My kids need help with their homework when I'm trying to finish writing a blog post.

HOW TO STOP EATING YOUR FEELINGS

○   Desire: I want chocolate.

If a dog drools, do you try and put the drool back in their mouth? Or do you just get a paper towel and wipe it up?

You wipe it up, right? It's fruitless to try and put the drool back in their mouth (and kinda gross too.)

It's the same thing with desire. Once the desire is there, trying to put it back in is fruitless. But that's what we're doing when we resist our desire. Whether you're hankering for Zagnuts or Zinfandel, once the desire is there, resisting it won't make it go away.

Resisting creates a battle of cognitive dissonance within you. I want it / I don't want it. That dissonance amps up the anxiety. And increased anxiety feeds the desire for whatever substance you're jonesing for, in order to make the anxiety go away. It's a vicious cycle. ("Darn you drool!!!!")

There's a lesser-known part of Pavlov's experiment. Once the trigger-desire pattern was established (bell ⇒ drool), Pavlov also wanted to see what would happen when he rang the bell but did NOT bring the dogs food.

Naturally, at first, they still had the patterned response. Bell ⇒ drool ⇒ no food. But over time, the dogs learned that the bell no longer meant that food was coming. So they gradually unlearned the patterned response.

Just like doggie brains, our brains can be trained too. Desire can be unlearned. But first you gotta look that desire in the face and question if it's true.

Imperfect Brains

"Holy Mother of Pearl!" I exclaimed as I (no joke) jumped fifteen feet in the air away from the snake.

My daughter and I were walking the dogs when I noticed the snake out of the corner of my eye. We live in Florida and the poisonous Cottonmouth snake is common where we live. I was worried that the dogs would spook it and cause it to strike at them.

Thank goodness I saved the dogs from a painful bite and mortal injury!

Then my daughter said, *"Uhm, where's the snake?"*

"It's right therrrwhhaaaaa??!?!??"

I was pointing right at the snake so Annie could see it. (And avoid it! Hello!?!)

Except I was pointing at a stick.

Are you serious? I just freaked out over a stick?

Sigh.

My heart was racing. My palms were sweaty. I had all the physical reactions to a real snake, and I was so ready to fight or flight my way outta there, dragging my daughter along with me.

But what was going on inside my head was NOT REAL.

We do this all the time. While it's easy to realize my thoughts about a really big scary snake were not true when it turns out to be a stick, other false thoughts can be harder to spot.

Your brain is imperfect. It is going to have thoughts that are not always helpful. Like "I want crackers even though I'm not hungry."

Brains have thoughts. That's what they do.

Yet we expect our brains to be perfect when we wish that we could "just get over our cravings" or never have the desire to eat when we're not hungry or just see "food as fuel."

Expecting your brain to be perfect is like expecting an infant to sleep through the night. You can expect that all you want. But you're likely to be disappointed. It's not the baby's fault that its stomach is too small to keep it full longer than a few hours. In the same way, it's not your brain's fault that it comes up with thoughts like, "I want chocolate at the end of a long day."

Just because you have a thought doesn't make it true, nor does it mean that you need to act on it. It also doesn't mean that you're bad or weak because you had that thought.

The human brain is really good at delegating repeated patterns to the lower brain because that saves energy. When something is delegated to the lower brain, that makes it beneath the surface of your awareness. Remember Hagrid the Croc? Just because you can't see it, doesn't mean it's not there.

When you feel a desire for sugar or snacks, it is simply your lower brain repeating the habit loop. When you've always had a snack at 4 p.m., your brain is working properly when it sends up a snack suggestion at 3:45. It doesn't mean you have no willpower. It's simply something you've taught your brain to expect so it puts that pattern on repeat.

It can be scary to feel a little out of control of desire when the lower brain is making demands to satisfy the craving. Sugar can create increasing desire because it provides an intense reward to the brain. Your brain wants to feel good! The more the reward, the more the desire.

So we find ourselves faced with these competing desires. The prefrontal cortex (planning) part of your brain wants to fit into the jeans you wore last year. On the other hand, the subconscious (habit) part of your brain says, "I need chocolate right now or I will literally die."

Instead of assuming all your thoughts are true, what if you looked at your thoughts with curiosity? Rather than blindly believing that you ACTUALLY want chocolate right now, you can think, *"Huh. That's interesting. My brain is telling me I want chocolate. Is that true, or is it simply a habit that I have accidentally trained my brain to ask for chocolate at this time of day? What do I really want right now?"*

The lower brain is the in-the-moment decision maker. If you haven't planned ahead with your planning part of the brain, the lower brain will win every argument in the moment. Ev-er-y time.

There are three options when you feel desire:

1) Act on it.

   Eat the cookie or pour the drink. This perpetuates the cycle.

2) Resist it.

   Push against it. This creates anxiety, which increases the desire. Desire + anxiety wears you down and eventually you cave, thus perpetuating the cycle.

3) Allow it.

   Don't resist the desire. Don't try to make it go away. Basically, allow your doggie brain to drool all over your mental sofa. Don't try to push the drool back into the dog's mouth. Observe the feeling in your body, but don't act on the desire.

The desire in itself is not harmful. It's not a problem. You can coexist with the desire as long as you're not trying to resist it. Resistance makes the desire go up.

We are so quick to want to get rid of the desire that we try to squish it. It's important to make room for both and give them both their due.

"What you resist, persists."
~Carl Jung

If you're thinking that *"Allowing desire sounds miserable!"*, you're not alone. That's exactly what I thought too. *"Great. I get to mentally (or maybe literally) drool all over the place, but I don't get to have my chocolate at the end? Who decided this was a good idea?!?"*

If you find yourself trying to resist the desire, it's only because you haven't learned how not to resist and how to allow it.

Learning to allow and sit with the discomfort of desire is something you can learn. When you learn how to allow an urge, you realize that the desire, the urge, is completely harmless. The only time it becomes a problem is when you act on it or resist it.

Just Follow Your L.I.S.T.

What does allowing even mean?

We are so used to resisting, it's hard to imagine what "allowing" even means. We have been conditioned to white-knuckle it.

Think of it this way:

Imagine you're in a river and there's a waterfall downstream.

1) You can swim with the current and go over the waterfall. That's acting on the desire.

2) You can swim against the current, get tired out, and eventually get swept over the waterfall. That's resistance or trying to use willpower.

3) Or you can swim to the side where the current isn't so strong and watch the water go by. That's allowing the urge.

The more you can be present with yourself and the desire, the more you can realize, "I'm okay right now, in this second." As soon as you start thinking into the future, "I don't know if I can hold out" that's when resistance comes in.

What would it be like to make all your feelings and desires okay?

Use the acronym L.I.S.T. to help you allow your feelings and cravings.

1) Look for it
2) Identify it
3) Surrender to it
4) Track it

1) LOOK FOR IT

You can expect the desire to come. It's a given.

Your brain is simply operating on the old habit cycle that you've taught it. It's like knowing the tide is coming in. No matter where you build your sandcastle, you can still expect the tide to come.

There's nothing wrong with you when that desire comes. You can expect it to faithfully show up around the same time each day because you've taught your brain that a reward is coming. It just sends up the signal, "Hey, it's reward time."

I used to feel like a failure when I would predictably feel a desire for wine around 5 p.m. "Something's wrong with me!" But it was just my brain doing exactly what I had taught it to do. As soon as I released the judgment of myself, seeing the desire come in at 5 p.m. was just something I expected and accepted.

Expecting cravings to go away is like asking a running coach to teach you how to not get tired when running a marathon. If a marathon runner said to themselves, "I feel tired. I must be doing this wrong," they'd never finish a race.

So step one is don't judge yourself for feeling the desire for a treat. It's just your brain following the pattern it has learned!

There's always the option to indulge in the craving. But just like the runner, there's also an option to keep going another minute, or another five minutes and see what happens.

Lean into allowing it.

2) IDENTIFY IT

Plan to allow yourself the treat you desire. But before actually having it, take a moment to look inward and name what you're feeling. *"I'm feeling angry that Ted didn't send the report on time so then I had to hustle at the end of the day."* or *"I'm feeling lonely because Sue left town yesterday."*

Just allow it to be there. It's okay to have feelings! They're normal. You're normal! And you are strong enough to feel them fully.

Next, get connected to the feeling in your body. What are the sensations you're feeling?

If you were to explain this feeling to an alien who had no concept of feelings, how would you describe what it feels like?

- tightness in my chest
- tension in my shoulders
- heaviness in my stomach

The more you describe the sensations you feel, the more you realize you can survive it. A feeling is just a vibration in your body.

Try writing it out.

Sometimes I feel like my thoughts are so embarrassing and shameful that I REALLY don't ever want anyone else to see them. So I have a note in an app on my phone (labeled "Note" so that no one would know it's my personal thoughts) where I can write out what's in my head when my thoughts are yelling at me.

It is amazing how powerful that simple act is. Just getting them out of my head helps me look at my thoughts with curiosity rather than judgment and think, "Well that all makes sense now. No wonder I'm feeling upset."

Maybe get curious and ask yourself a few questions.

1) Where are you hanging out in your thoughts?
   - In the past, ruminating about something that happened in the day?
   - In the future wondering if/when you'll have a treat or feel stressed about not having one?

Just notice.

2) What's the role you're playing in the story you're telling yourself?

- Often, we play the victim when we're thinking of wanting a treat. "I had a really long day! I deserve it."

- And then we play the villain in our mind the next day. "I can't believe I did that again."

- How can you be the hero in your own story?

3) What's this urge or desire actually about? What are you avoiding?

- Often, we're avoiding a feeling.

- Don't judge yourself if having a treat has become a way for you to practice self-care. Instead recognize that we've been taught to go on this external hunt to look for something outside ourselves to feel better.

- If you can't write it out, talk it out. Keep an audio journal in an app on your phone. Call a friend. Talk to your plants. They're much better listeners than cats.

4) Will a treat really address what's underneath the desire (from #3)? How will it NOT solve that tension?

- Sometimes we realize that having a treat will actually make the reason we want a treat (like fatigue or stress) worse.

5) What are reasons why I DON'T want it?

- Sometimes just reminding yourself of the reasons why you DON'T want it in the long run can give you pause and let your conscious mind have a voice in the conversation.

6) How can I be the parent to my toddler brain that wants a pacifier in the moment?
   - The subconscious mind is a lot like a toddler. Imagine you gave a toddler a piece of candy every day at 5 p.m.
   - Then one day you decide, "Nope. No more candy."
   - The toddler still wants it and will probably throw a fit when he doesn't get it.
   - That's not a problem. You, as the parent, know what's better for the toddler so you can patiently ride out the tantrum.
   - Your subconscious mind is exactly like a toddler expecting its 5 p.m. candy.

7) What do I REALLY deserve?
   - Sometimes the reason we tell ourselves that we want a treat is because "I deserve it."
   - That feels true in the moment.
   - But if you step back and ask yourself, "What do I REALLY deserve?" that can give your conscious mind a chance to say things like:
     o I deserve to feel great in my body tomorrow.
     o I deserve to go to bed without feeling overly full.
     o I deserve to feel proud of myself.
     o I deserve to keep my word to myself.
     o I deserve to know that I am making progress and not sabotaging myself.

It's okay when your brain sends up the thought "I deserve it" but that doesn't mean you have to believe it without asking questions.

3) SURRENDER TO IT

Surrender Technique A:

If you're a person of faith, here's a way to describe what it's like to allow your feelings or allow a craving.

Proactively let go and release what you're feeling to God or the Universe. Remind yourself:

"I am safe. I can be free to feel my feelings because I am safe to let go, and I know that I am completely held. This is already working out for me."

Let God handle all your feelings for you.

Surrender Technique B:

Imagine how you would respond if your child walked into the room with tears in their eyes. Not the "I'm injured" kind of tears. But the "My feelings are hurt and I just need to cry about it" kind of tears.

How would you treat your child?

Now imagine that the feeling you have is just like your child who needs to talk it out a little. Whether you're feeling a craving or stress or anxiety, how can you look at the feeling like an entity in itself and treat it with kindness and understanding?

Surrender Technique C:

Another strategy is to look inward into your body.

Sit quietly for a minute.

Try and locate the feeling in your body.

- Where is it?
  - Stomach? Shoulders? Chest?
- How would you describe the sensation?
  - Tightness? Burning? Heaviness?
- If you could give this feeling a shape, what shape would it be?
  - A spiky ball? A blob? Like a gas?
- What color would it be?
  - Yellow? Brownish green? Gray?

Address this feeling / shape as if you could speak to it inside your mind.

"Thank you for being here. I see you. I honor you. You're allowed to be here."

1. [To the feeling] *"If you could speak, what would you say?"*
   a. Just listen. What comes up?
2. [To the feeling] *"What is your purpose here?"*
   a. Often the feeling is there to protect you.
3. [To the feeling] *"What message do you have for me?"*
   a. This can be really enlightening.

Thank the feeling for being there and just imagine that you are sitting next to it on a bench. Just sit there next to it. You don't have to make it go away. Just be with it.

After a minute or two, what is the shape and color of the feeling? Has it changed?

If you feel inspired to do so, try journaling about what you experienced and what you learned from the feeling.

> ## TAKE IT FURTHER
>
> For a print out of surrender techniques to help you handle emotional hunger without turning to food, go to https://confidentbody.coach/book/ to download your book extras.

Surrender Technique D:

[If you're not a fan of water or swimming, you might want to skip this one.]

Imagine you're in a body of water and you're trying to stay afloat.

Your difficult feelings or desire for the craving are the water.

Instead of resisting, simply let go and allow yourself to slip under water, surrendering to the feeling of it.

You breathe in and you find that you can breathe underwater and survive within it.

The important piece is the surrendering. LEAN INTO the feeling.

You don't act on the craving, you simply allow yourself to FEEL it.

Just try five minutes at a time to build up that muscle and prove to yourself that you can handle a craving or a negative feeling.

Please remember that everything is an experiment. If something works, great. Keep it.

If something doesn't work, great. Tweak it.

Everything is helping you and there's never a reason to feel guilty or shame yourself. All wins and losses are helping you learn more about yourself and that's the win in the long run!

"Most of our suffering comes from resisting what is already here, particularly our feelings. All any feeling wants is to be welcomed, touched, allowed. It wants attention. It wants kindness.
If you treated your feelings with as much love as you treated your dog or your cat or your child, you'd feel as if you were living in heaven every day of your sweet life."
~Geneen Roth

4) TRACK IT

You can't take away a reward from your brain and expect it to be just fine without a replacement reward.

Keep a tracker of days that you've gone through these prompts as a mental reward.

Give yourself visible credit for the work you're doing!

Use a jar of marbles or a tracking sheet to give yourself the win of seeing progress. After five minutes of allowing the desire, put a marble in a clear jar or mark it on the sheet.

It's important to be able to see it. Having it on a note in your phone doesn't work as well because it's not as visible. This creates a mental reward.

Remember, your brain got a reward from having the treat, so you've got to give it a replacement reward for NOT having the treat, otherwise you'll have a mutiny in your brain.

Aim to fill up the jar or the tracking sheet over the course of a few months.

You still get to have what you desire, just put it off for five minutes and really lean into what that desire FEELS like.

Soften toward it. Welcome it in.

Get curious about it.

The skill is being able to watch yourself think and not react. You're the witness watching yourself have the urge. Observe those sentences with peace and curiosity and fascination and try not to get wrapped up in the drama of it.

The desire is completely harmless unless you react to it or fight it. Your brain is not trying to hurt you by bringing these thoughts up. It's trying to survive. It's trying to save you from pain.

You may not be able to do this the first time or the first twenty times you try. I didn't. But you can learn it with practice. Watch yourself have a desire and not act on it. It's very different from resisting it and wishing it wasn't there.

Three steps forward and two steps back is really normal!!

Imagine it like this:

Learning to surf takes hours to learn. Every wipe out you have before getting up on that board looks like failure, but you're actually learning. Each failure is not actually failure. Each wipe out is a CRUCIAL part of the process of getting to a place where you feel more confident and can stand on the board successfully.

Each time you try to allow an urge and feel tense because you're resisting or find yourself acting on it, that's okay. Keep at it. You're learning a skill.

NOTE: Please don't think of this as simply resisting and will-powering your way to thirty days without sugar or a dry January. Ultimately that will only increase your desire. Do not try and white knuckle it. Allow the urge to be there.

What if you did an experiment?

Maybe give yourself a week or five days.

"For the next five days, before I indulge in whatever I am craving, I'll take five minutes to do this exercise and get curious about the feeling in my body."

Then after five minutes you can have the treat you're craving.

Could be interesting to see what comes up!

Experiencing negative feelings and "getting down" is a normal and expected part of life. Sure, it helps to proactively maintain a positive mindset, but life is not meant to be happy all the time. We are meant to have a balance of positive and negative emotions. That's part of this beautiful, brutal, magnificent, excruciating, wondrous ride we call "being human."

I have a theory that before your soul or my soul came to incarnate as who we are today, some sort of wisdom inside us knew that life would be ALL the things. All the ups AND the downs. And in our soul's wisdom, we said "Yes! Sign me up for that!"

"My aim isn't to feel happy. It is to feel everything."
~Glennon Doyle

But What If I Fail?

Let me tell you, when I first tried this, the voice of fear inside my heart was fah-reak-ing out. She was yelling, whining, moaning, saying, "But what if I screw this up? What if I fail?" The perfectionist inside me was sooooo not into this because I was terrified that I would suck at it and fall off the wagon...hard.

We are afraid to fail because of what that failure would MEAN.

But what if you could make it mean something other than you're a sucky human that is destined to wallow in failure?

For me, "What if I fail?" loomed large and in charge in my thoughts. Until I decided to choose a new thought that also felt true.

"I can figure this out. This whole process is about learning, and I am pretty good at learning new things."

That was the thought I tuned into when the desire came in strong and hot at 5:01 p.m. each night. I'd go a few days really jamming on that thought-redirect, and then something would disrupt my patterns and I'd forget it for a while.

Be smarter than me.

Find a new, more empowering thought than "What if I fail?" and write it down. Sticky note it to your desk, your mirror, your forehead. Give yourself the best shot at filling your head with thoughts that lead to positive feelings. Because those positive feelings lead to intentional actions that lead to results that just might blow away your expectations of what you thought you were capable of.

You've got this.

I Think I'll Feel Deprived

Feeling deprived comes from restriction. That's not what we're doing here. Make a plan to allow the desire AND to have the cookies or the chips. It sounds counterintuitive, but allowing the desire teaches you that you are just fine and over time that reduces the desire's power over you.

Here's a way to implement this:

PLAN AHEAD.

Have a meeting with (1) you now, (2) your future self who is in the moment, tired from a long day, wanting the food you desire, and (3) future you the day after the food eating event. Plan how much you'll have, knowing that future you in the moment will want it.

You can't rely on yourself to do what you want in the future without using your conscious brain for planning. Plan on what your subconscious habit brain is going to say in the moment and have an answer for it.

Ask yourself what objections your brain brings up in the moment when you want potato chips or ice cream. You know they're coming and you're ready and you have an answer for them, so you don't let them drive your action.

1. How might the three of you compromise on a plan for how much you want to have in the moment?
2. How might you anticipate that the urge to have more is coming?
3. What helps you be present with that desire when it comes in and allow it rather than resist it?

Have an honest conversation with yourself about what you're willing to commit to, what you're not, and have a collaborative conversation around what the commitment will be.

Consider all those components.

If things go exactly as planned, great! High five all three of yo-selves!

When things don't go the way you planned, reconvene and figure out why. Use curiosity, not condemnation. Be gentle. No judgment. Make sure your commitment honors you and serves to build your self-esteem versus being a way to break yourself down.

This Sounds Like A Lot Of Work

Yes! It does take effort. That's a GOOD thing!

Not thinking and not working is how you got to this point in the first place. The brain wants to efficiently delegate thoughts and patterns to the subconscious mind because that's EASY.

It's like saying, "You know, I think my four-year-old is mature enough to be in charge of dinner." Then you give him free reign in the kitchen and act surprised when the spatula is on fire because he left it on the burner and he's crying because he sliced his finger with the knife.

You already know what happens when you allow your brain to delegate the thought-action pattern of "When I get home from the office, I reach for a bag of chips." You get that automatic, Pavlovian response that makes you feel out of control.

SO WHAT if it's work?

You can't sit on the couch while your four-year-old burns the kitchen down and say, "It'll be fine. He'll figure it out." You've got to stand up and DO SOMETHING.

That's what this is all about. You're proactively pulling that previously delegated thought up out of the basement of your subconscious and into the light of day.

It's natural to think that urges and desires are something you want to avoid. It can feel uncomfortable to just allow it. However, what if you could view these moments in a different light? What if every time you feel an urge and allow it, that's a positive thing because it means that it's an opportunity for you to get in reps when it counts?

If your goal is to eventually lift 50 pounds, you'd start with the little two pound weights. Then build up to the five and then the ten pound weights. You're building the muscle of being willing to feel any emotion, one rep at a time.

Feeling an urge is a sign that "it's working!"

Just like learning to surf. It takes hours of practice. But once you know how, you know how forever. Falling off and falling off again is normal when learning to surf.

It's not failing. It's learning.

It's the same with learning to allow desire. Keep getting back up. It's absolutely worth it. Your freedom is on the other side.

What Does Success Look Like?

Some clients tell me that they'll feel like they've succeeded when they "get over their old habits."

Waiting until you no longer feel any urges, desires, cravings, or temptations before you can feel successful is hurting you in the long run.

Let's look at this from a different angle. Let's say you wanted to learn to play tennis. In order to learn and get better at tennis, you'd likely take some lessons and begin to improve. At the same time, you'd probably still have some bad habits from time to time, like bad footwork or taking your racquet back too late, etc.

Nevertheless, as you practice more, you can see that you're improving, and you've come a long way. Those bad habits are still there sometimes, but you're working on them.

At what point in your tennis journey have you "succeeded"?

The truth is that you're succeeding all along the way in lots of ways that add up to your significant transformation as a tennis player.

Conquering cravings and urges is similar. There's no finish line. You're succeeding in little and big ways all the time! Don't put your happiness and your success "out there" beyond some arbitrary marker. That's like trying to chase the horizon. It's always a little out of reach.

There really is no "finish line" for when you'll "be a success" as a tennis player. It's a practice. A discipline. It's about improving upon who you were yesterday rather than reaching some external benchmark. Learning to allow cravings is the same thing.

CHAPTER 10
HOW TO MOTIVATE

Kathleen was a diet pro. She'd done Weight Watchers, Keto, Paleo, Whole 30, Isagenix, and I think she even tried going vegan for a little while. After working together for several weeks, she was frustrated.

> Kathleen: *This should be easy by now!*
>
> Me: *Tell me more.*
>
> Kathleen: *I've done so many diets. I know WHAT to do. I just don't do it. You'd think that by now I'd get the hang of things.*
>
> *But every time I do well for a few weeks and then I have an early work meeting, or my son Kyle has a late basketball game, or we go away on a long weekend. I get a little bit out of the routine, and I stop planning ahead because I'm tired and always trying to catch up.*
>
> *Pretty soon, three weeks have passed. I'm terrified of stepping on the scale and I'm right back where I started (or worse). I've lost my motivation.*

Ah, motivation. What is this magic elixir you speak of?

Merriam-Webster defines motivation as: a motivating force, stimulus, or influence.[29]

But what actually IS it?

Sometimes motivation can feel like trying to hold on to water. It's constantly slipping through the cracks between your fingers.

Can we get real for a second?

If you're relying on feeling motivated to get you through, that's always going to run out eventually. Motivation is a feeling. And just like any other feeling (happy, sad, frustrated, relaxed, etc.) feelings come and go.

Instead, think ahead to the inevitable times when that feeling of motivation will wane. Expect it.

What are you going to do when that happens?

How can you draw on the strengths you already have to help you through?

As Kathleen and I dug a little deeper, I asked what patterns she noticed when she felt "off track."

> Me: *So you said you know *what* to do in order to help you get back on track. You just don't do it. What gets in the way?*
>
> Kathleen: *Planning ahead is a lot of work.*
>
> Me: *"A lot of work." Okay, let's look at other areas of your life. When you kids were small, was taking care of them a lot of work?*
>
> Kathleen: *Yes, sometimes.*
>
> Me: *What did you do when it got hard?*
>
> Kathleen: *I just kept going. They needed me.*

29 https://www.merriam-webster.com/dictionary/motivation

Me: *How about in your job? Are there ever times when it feels hard, or you don't feel like going to work that day?*
Kathleen: *I guess. Sure. But, you know, you just do it.*
Me: *So there were times when your boys were young that it was hard work to take care of them. Yet you chose to do it. It didn't really seem like a choice. Because caring for your children is part of your identity. It's who you ARE.*
In your profession, there are times when it feels like a lot of work. And yet you don't just skip a day when you feel like it because that's not what you do. It's not part of who you ARE.
Kathleen: *Hmmm. I see where you're going with this.*

Kathleen was the same person when she was taking care of her kids as she was when she was trying to diet. The difference was the story she was telling herself about when things got hard.

We think that motivation is about feeling excited to take action on the goals we want for ourselves. But it's not. Motivation is about what we do and how we think when things get hard.

There are things in life that we do, even when we don't feel motivated or excited to do them. We do them because it is just part of our belief system.

The person who says, *"I have to go to the gym today so I look good for my vacation to Hawaii next month"* has different beliefs about themselves than the person that thinks *"I go to the gym because I like how it makes me feel. I'm the kind of person who goes to the gym."*

When it's cold outside and you're tired from staying up late to finish a work project, rocking a bikini next month is not all that compelling. However, if you see exercise as a way to destress and feel good, you have a different motivation for getting out of bed.

When things get hard, a mom gets up in the night with her kids because it's part of who she is as a mom.

==> The key moment is when things get tough.

Setbacks in your work life or frustrating moments with your kids are normal. They're part of the job. You expect them and persevere through them.

And there will be setbacks in your weight loss journey too. It's normal.

Expect them.

The question is what will be your mindset when that happens?

What is the action you want to take when unexpected things get in the way of the habits you're trying to establish?

What would you need to believe about yourself in order to persevere through them?

How might you treat stumbles and setbacks in your weight loss journey in the same way that you treated a mess on the floor when your kid was potty training? (Okay, maybe that's a bad example. Potty training drove me crazy. Anyway, you get it.) How can you use the frustrating thing as evidence of "this is just part of the process" rather than as evidence for why you should quit?

Remember, you can level up your identity a little bit at a time. You don't have to jump from *"Planning ahead is hard"* to *"I'm the kind of person who makes meal plans every Sunday."*

Instead, look for little pieces of evidence along the way.

Look for evidence like... *"I can plan two nights a week." "I'm the kind of person who is willing to think ahead for how I might feel at 3 p.m. and make a plan for it." "I'm willing to plan out my snack today, and maybe tomorrow too."*

And of course, give yourself credit for what you've done already and little ways you're already leveling up!

I'll say it a hundred times if I have to: Giving yourself the chance to FEEL GOOD ABOUT YOURSELF is the fuel that keeps you going.

Thoughts That Destroy Motivation

When things get hard, the brain predictably sends up sneaky thoughts that snuff out the fire of motivation and resilience in the face of challenges. Be on the alert for them so you can be prepared to handle them.

Why Bother?

"I'm working so hard, but the scale is not moving. So why bother?"

Progress is the fuel that ignites the engine motivation. So when you're not seeing the progress you want on the scale, that's when motivation begins to wane.

However, asking yourself "Why bother?" makes you feel like the victim in your own story.

Take agency of your circumstances by owning your thoughts.

Turn that thought around to:

"I know the scale will change at some point. But it won't change if I give up on what I've been doing.

Spend time thinking about all the amazing things you're doing for your body, rather than getting upset about what's not happening on your own made-up timeline.

When you say yes to one thing, you say no to something else.

In this case, saying yes to the old way you used to eat, that's saying no to the new benefits you've been enjoying.

You can accomplish anything…if you just keep going and you release your grip on the timeline.

> *"Success and failure are on the same road.*
> *Success is just further down that road."*
> *~Susie Moore*

It's understandable to want the result to be faster than it is. But you only hurt yourself when you say, "This isn't working." How long have you been doing it? Two weeks? Five months? How long did it take you to gain the weight? Five years? Ten years?

Don't give the problem a year and the solution a week. Ask yourself if you're focusing more on the energy of the problem than the energy of solution. It's unkind to give yourself ten years to gain the weight and ten days, or even ten weeks, to lose it.

You can be generous to yourself and generous to the solution. Give yourself time and space so that you can keep going even when results aren't happening as fast as you'd like.

Changing habits is playing the long game. If you want to change your habits, change your thoughts. If you want to change your thoughts, practice new thoughts. If you want to change faster, get in more reps.

- Practice your personal mantras twice a day for thirty days.
- Practice looking for ways you are disinterested in over-eating. Schedule your practice time. Bundle it with something you already do regularly. Practice the thought.
- Practice looking for things you love about healthy eating / living / exercise. Plan time to do the thinking. Bundle it. Get in the reps.
- Write down what you've learned. Keep a log. Keep a learning journal. Write it down some more.
- Imagine 100 reps. How many days will it take to get in 100 mental reps? 200 reps? Mark that on the calendar to set your mental expectations.

When expectations aren't being met, it doesn't mean to quit doing amazing things for yourself. It just means your timeline is delayed.

This Should Be Easy By Now

If you've been at this a while, planning your meals, eating more veggies, exercising on the regular, you might be thinking *"I am ready for this process to be my natural way of life without so much effort."* That's understandable. We live in a world where we don't have to be patient for much at all.

We think that our goal is to get to a place where *"Eventually it'll be easy. I just want to not have to think about it so much."*

Telling yourself that story in your mind ends up making you feel worse when it doesn't start to happen as soon as you'd like.

Here's what you can expect instead:

When you make a change, the mental drama will come up.

EXPECT IT.

It's okay. It's just your brain sending up thoughts because your subconscious mind is a little freaked out by change. This is NORMAL. Nothing has gone wrong.

Remember how patterns of thought can be like ski tracks in the snow? The more you practice an old thought, the deeper that groove is in your brain.

Comparatively speaking, your new patterns haven't had much opportunity to become your "natural way of life without so much effort."

So it's still gonna take proactive effort for a while to groove in those new tracks in your brain.

If you were to take a class in molecular biology or learn a new language, at what point would you expect it to be easy? When exactly do you become fluent in the new language?

In the same way, you are learning to train your brain in a different way and hone in the practice on new habits of thought. Managing your thoughts and emotions is like becoming fluent in a new language. It takes time and practice.

Part of the problem with diets is that they don't allow us to feel good until we've reached the finish line. That's where the feeling of impatience comes from. Diets don't teach you how to be grateful for how you showed up each day, however imperfect it was.

Stop and take a moment to look at how far you've come.

- How many pounds have you lost already? That in itself is a HUGE win!!! If you never changed another thing, that's something to feel proud of.

- You are making positive choices during the day that help your body feel healthier than it was. That's a win too!
- You're probably also drinking more water and getting in some movement. More wins!

So before you go feeling like all is lost, give yourself as much credit and high fives as possible for the fact that you've taken steps to change your life.

For real.

Nothing can erase that.

Unless you give up.

It is in those small moments when it feels hard, you can learn to have a better conversation in your head. Instead of telling yourself, "This isn't working," tell yourself *It's okay. This is all just a learning process. I can figure this out.*

How can you start to allow yourself to feel good today about what you ARE doing each day, no matter how small?

I Still Have So Far To Go

Sometimes weight loss can feel overwhelming. Especially if you feel like you're currently pretty far from your goal.

When you have a big goal you're trying to achieve, looking at it all at once can be intimidating and demoralizing.

It's like staring up a mountain and thinking, *I need to get to the top of THAT?!?"*

Remember the analogy of rolling a rock up a hill to overcome activation energy?

YOU ARE A MIRACLE

Whether we're talking about tackling a big work project, hiking a mountain, or losing weight, it can be beneficial to break the goal down into smaller steps and mini milestones.

If you were trying to run a marathon, would you start out with a fifteen mile run? Hopefully not. You'd start with smaller runs to build up your strength and endurance and take it one week, one day, one mile at a time.

So instead of looking at ALL the weight you want to lose, what if you only focused on the next three pounds? How would that feel in terms of overwhelm versus feasibility?

If you have a big goal in front of you, just focus on the next step. The next choice.

> *"Nobody trips over mountains. It is the small pebble that causes you to stumble. Pass all the pebbles in your path, and you will find you have crossed the mountain."*
> *~Author Unknown*

Hacks For Kickstarting Your Motivation

Motivation is all about how you think about your efforts, your progress, and your success. Use these mindsets to help you strengthen your motivation and resilience when life inevitably throws curveballs your way.

Keep Your Tank Full

"If only I had more willpower, then I could...."

"I really struggle with X because I have NO willpower."

Why is it that we treat willpower like the magic pill? We never have enough of it, but if we did, then we'd be perfect. We'd be able to resist the temptation, get the workout done, and never be short with our spouse or yell at our kids.

Here's the thing about willpower: It's like a muscle. It can get stronger if you use it more. It can get weaker if you never use it. And it most certainly can get tired and worn out.

I like to think of willpower like a gas tank. Let's say on a normal day, you start the day with a full tank of willpower. All sorts of things draw "gas" from your willpower tank.

Decisions of any kind draw on your willpower tank. Deciding what to wear in the morning draws on your willpower tank. (That's why people like Steve Jobs famously always wore the same thing. So they didn't have to decide.) Deciding whether or not to work out. Deciding what to eat. Deciding what not to eat draws on your willpower tank. Deciding whether or not to attend a social event.

Frustrations and stress most definitely draw on your willpower tank. Traffic. A concern over your child's grade in school. Having a busy day. Needing to take the dog to the vet. Worrying (about anything). All of these things use up willpower.

Fatigue uses up willpower as well. Let's say you got one less hour of sleep last night. You're already starting the day with a willpower tank that's ¾ full (or less.) Is it any wonder that we crave sweets and carbs more when we're tired?

Many of us start the day out strong with wonderful intentions. The day goes well till maybe around 3-5 p.m. Then it's like we have a completely different brain than the one we woke up with. We negotiate with ourselves later in the day. Then it feels like we just can't reign it in and the diet is blown. Again.

It is harder to make good choices when you're tired.

It's because your willpower tank is near empty by that time of day! All the little decisions, stresses, and normal activities of life have drained your willpower down to almost nothing so that you don't have the stamina to say no to the chips or cookies or take-out for dinner at the end of the day.

So what do you do about it? How do you stack the willpower deck in our favor?

Make fewer decisions.

Take deciding out of your day whenever you can.

- Plan ahead for what you're going to eat.
  - There are lots of different ways to meal plan. Many folks plan dinner meals for weeknights and leave themselves flexibility on weekends. Others start the day (with a full willpower tank) and decide what they'll eat for the rest of the day in the morning. (Don't worry. I've got you covered. There's a whole chapter on meal planning later in the Imperfect Toolbox.)
- Plan for afternoon or late-night snack time.
  - When you feel tempted in the evening and you know that your willpower is already low, plan ahead for that time. Have a snack ready to go. Plan an activity to keep your mind busy. Do what you can to prepare. When you know that it's not your fault that your willpower is lower, you can prepare for it.

- Decide when you're going to work out.
  - Remove the "if" and replace it with "when".
  - Decide what kind of workout you want to do. Plan for these things when you have a fresh willpower tank.
- Work out earlier in the day when your willpower tank is full so you're more likely to be able to get over the activation energy to get going.
- Do little things during the day to relieve stress.
  - Go for a walk. Meditate for one minute. Take three deep breaths.

Motivation is all about overcoming resistance to do the thing you want in the long term vs. going with what's easy in the moment. Lower the resistance and your motivation increases.

Just Start

Have you ever listened to a motivational speaker? I confess, I love those kinds of talks. I get all fired up and I'm like, "Yeah! Let's storm the castle!"

However, I also know that about a day and a half after I've been all pumped up from listening to a great motivational speaker, my life gets busy and all those ideas and resolutions for change get buried under the regular detritus of life.

The whole premise behind motivational speakers is that feeling leads to action. And it's true. We walked through the S.T.E.A.R. model of how our thoughts create feelings which lead to actions and actions lead to results.

And...the opposite is also true.

Action can influence feelings. Sit on the couch for three days straight and you'll feel pretty low. Go for a walk at the end of a long day and you feel a little better than you did on the car ride home.

Actions make us feel. Feelings make us act. The mind body connection is a two-way street.

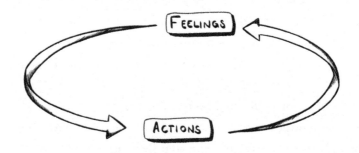

When you wash a car, how do you hold the hose? You put your finger over the nozzle of the hose to concentrate the water, right? Concentrating the water pressure makes the hose more powerful.

In weight loss, concentrate your action on a small area where you know you can make a difference.

You can't always control how motivated you'll feel, but you can control your choice to take tiny actions. Even little actions can change the way you feel and increase your motivation.

When you rely on how you feel as the deciding factor of what you do, you'll be a slave to it. Your outcomes will be as unreliable as your feelings. (Unless you're proactively choosing your thoughts, of course!)

Action generates more action. Don't wait to expect to want to take action by waiting for motivation to strike. Create a position of strength by making a tiny habit which does not require much willpower. A tiny action is a powerful way to get you rolling toward feeling motivated.

Have you ever felt tired after work, but when you mustered up the energy to go for a walk you felt better afterward? It's a funny contradiction that we feel "too tired" to walk, but walking makes us feel more energetic!

Sometimes starting with an action before you "feel like it" can help your mind and heart feel more motivated to do it.

Strive For Imperfection

When motivation is on the fritz, lower your expectations of yourself. Don't try to be perfect. Try to be IMPERFECT!

Try using the sentence "Can I just....XYZ?"

- Can I just have a side salad with my pizza?
- Can I just have two handfuls of candy instead of four?
- Can I just split the ice cream with my partner instead of having a whole serving?
- Can I just leave a little bit of wine in the glass and not finish it?

The sentence "Can I just...." Helps you remember that even a little positive choice is a vote for yourself.

It's a vote for saying, "Yeah, I can do hard things."

Little by little "Can I just do X" begins to change your mindset around those little, and sometimes bigger things, that you can do for yourself. It begins to build up evidence to prove to your brain that you are worth it.

The Most Powerful Three-Letter Word

One word can be the difference you need today.

Just three letters.

Y.E.T.

What does it feel like to tell yourself "This isn't working" versus "This isn't working ....yet."

You're doing the work.

You're showing up for yourself consistently.

Now all you need is practice.

It isn't working....YET.

Keep going.

Make It Mean Something

In 1666, more than half of London burned to the ground in the Great Fire of London. The city was in shambles. King Charles II commissioned architect Sir Christopher Wren to rebuild the city, include the famous St. Paul's Cathedral.

(Coincidentally, Sir Christopher Wren also built the famous Wren Building at my alma mater, The College William and Mary. But I digress...)

One day in 1671, as Sir Christopher oversaw the rebuilding of St. Paul's Cathedral, he saw three bricklayers on a scaffold.

As the first one was crouched down, and he asked the man, *"What are you doing?"* The bricklayer replied, *"Oy. I'm a bricklayer. I'ma cuttin' stone so it'll fit a certain shape and support this here wall."*

The second bricklayer was half standing, working hard at his task. When Sir Christopher asked, *"What are you doing?"* He replied, *"I'm a builder. I'm building a wall to support my family."*

Sir Christopher nodded. He knew it was admirable to work to support one's family. But then his eye was caught by the third bricklayer who stood proud and tall. This man clearly had a purpose.

Sir Christopher asked this man, *"What are you doing, sir?"* The man replied reverently, *"I am a cathedral builder. I am helping Sir Christopher Wren build the great Saint Paul's Cathedral to the Almighty."*

These three men were building the same wall, doing the same work, with three very different perspectives.

It's a good lesson. The attitude we bring to the task at hand makes all the difference. The meaning and purpose we attach to the work and challenges we endure can be the difference between a passing effort easily forgotten and the kind of work that leaves legacies.

How long have you struggled with your weight? So many of us have been battling our weight, and body image, for yeeeeeears. If not a lifetime.

Because of that, many of us have a story in our brains that says, "I can't lose weight" or "losing weight is ALWAYS a struggle for me" or "Why is this so freaking hard?"

Those stories feel really true. They make sense.

And yet, that story doesn't serve you. Frankly, you deserve a better story in your brain. One with meaning.

How can you look at your struggle as a gift? I know, I know. Bear with me for a second.

What if you could make your struggle with weight mean something powerful and deeply beautiful and meaningful to you?

For example:

- *"Because I have struggled with my weight, I will know how to help my daughter if and when she has similar issues. I will be better prepared to be what she needs, when she needs me."*

- *"Because I have struggled with my weight for so long, figuring this out will blow my mind of what I believe I am capable of. It will shift my identity around what I believe I can do. I wonder what else it will empower me to achieve?"*

- *"Because I have struggled with my weight, I can use this as an opportunity to have more compassion and empathy with others who are struggling with things I don't struggle with. Just because our challenges are not exactly the same, the experience of struggle is the same. I can be a good friend, or resource, or support to someone else who is suffering."*

How can you tell yourself a better story about your struggle? How is the challenge of it making you stronger? More compassionate? More prepared to help someone else? More of who you want to be in the world?

We don't admire perfect people. (Still not a thing.) We admire people who have gone through something, struggled, and been imperfect, and found something within themselves to be resilient and stronger than the challenges they faced. How can you make your journey mean something more to you?

"Nothing splendid has ever been achieved except by those who dared believe that something inside them was superior to the circumstances."
~*Bruce Barton*

A Visit From Your Future

Everyone gets discouraged sometimes. We feel tired and wonder if we'll ever reach our goals. Not every day is going to be perfect.

Everyone needs a pick-me-up from time to time, and not all of us have a cheerleader or a coach on the sidelines helping us remember how amazing we are. (By the way, you ARE amazing!)

When you find yourself feeling down, give this visualization a try.

It's five years from now.

You've lost the weight and you've been living at your comfortable weight for quite some time.

You have a positive relationship with food, and you actively appreciate your body for the amazing miracle it is.

Future you has been where you are now, and they navigated their way through it. Future-you is wise and patient and encouraging.

What would your future self say to you as encouragement to help you regain perspective when current-you steps on the scale and feels discouraged?

If future-you were to put their arm around your shoulders and tell you exactly what you need to hear in this moment, what would they say?

Success Is Like Bamboo

It can be so easy to get discouraged when you're not seeing the results you're hoping for. Even though you may intellectually know that plateaus, stalls, and ups and downs are normal, it is still easy to get discouraged sometimes.

When your motivation is low, think of Chinese bamboo.

The bamboo tree, like any plant, takes water and time for it to grow. But after the first year, there are no shoots to be seen. The roots are creating their foundation underground.

In fact, bamboo shoots don't come up for FIVE YEARS. Imagine how a gardener might feel after five years of tending and nurturing a garden with no visible growth to show for it! All that time, the bamboo tree is growing its foundational system of roots that will support it once it grows.

Then something amazing happens.

When the shoots do appear above ground, they grow up to eighty feet in just six weeks!

Success can be like that sometimes. It can feel like you're not seeing results when in fact the work you're doing is having important foundational effects on your mindset and your habits.

So give yourself some credit and patience to build your foundation for solid growth.

Exercise Motivation

Change The Way You Think About It

A lot of times clients will tell me *"I need to exercise more. When I force myself to actually do it, I always feel better afterward. It's just getting myself to do it that's the hard part. How do I remember that I like exercise when I don't want to do it?"*

We often think we don't like exercise because it's hard. Sometimes we use exercise to make up for overeating. When you're punishing yourself for something, it's no wonder that you don't like it!

Exercise doesn't have to be painful, and it should never be a punishment. Exercise doesn't even have to be "hard" for it to be useful.

The journey needs to be enjoyable, otherwise you won't like living at the destination.

What we focus on expands in our awareness.

If you focus on "I *should* exercise, but I don't like it," then the only thing you'll think about is the pain and dread of exercise.

Imagine an old-fashioned set of scales.

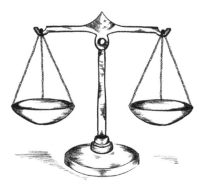

On one side is what you want in the moment (stay in bed, relax in front of the tv, etc.) and on the other side is what you want long term (a healthy body, feeling confident, etc.). The goal is to give more positive emotional weight to the side of the scale that you want long term rather than what you want in the moment.

The trick is to teach your brain to WANT to exercise and to like it, rather than only focusing on the result. You've got to learn to love the process if you want to be able to enjoy the result.

Since you can choose where to focus your attention, you can look for what's fun about exercise or focus on the good feeling that you like experiencing when you're finished. Focus on what you love about the habits you're trying to adopt and what you don't love about the habits you're trying to drop.

With exercise, the more you consciously, proactively think about how good you feel when you exercise, the more your brain will associate good feelings with it.

Here are some ideas:
- "I'll feel so good after....XYZ"
- "Even five minutes counts."
- "I'm lapping everyone on the couch."
- "Even though it can be hard to get started, I actually really DO feel better when I move."

At the end of the day, the best exercise for weight loss is the one you'll keep doing because you like it.

Maybe there's an opportunity for you to look into ways of moving your body that you don't normally consider exercise. For example, dancing, gardening, walking the dog, standing up and sitting back down again, playing with your kids....there are all kinds of ways to move your body that you don't normally associate with the pain of cardio or intense exercise.

⇒ What's one way to move your body that you could commit to doing consistently? Walk to the mailbox? Dance in the shower? Stretch before bed? It doesn't have to be huge. But you do have to proactively look for what you enjoy about it.

Once you have something that you can genuinely find that you enjoy about moving your body, here are some ideas for how to cultivate the feeling of liking exercise:

- Create space or a time in your day to proactively get quiet and think. (It doesn't have to be a long time. Two minutes is plenty.)
- Think about your last workout or movement of your body and how you felt afterward.
- Really bring that feeling into your body right now in this moment. Feel that uplifted feeling again.
- Smile. Appreciate your body for what it can do.
- Before bed, briefly try and think about that again so you're telling your mind what to remember while you're sleeping.

Conscious, proactive thought work is an important part of the process.

View Exercise As A Gift

When I played soccer in college, my least favorite conditioning was running. If someone was telling me to run, I resented it.

After college, I began to put on weight because I was sitting at a desk most of the day and not getting much exercise. I felt like I *should* go run, rather than actually wanting to.

Then a few years later, I hit a rough patch emotionally. My husband was deployed for military orders, we had two small kiddos and I worked a full-time job. We were in the middle of a very busy season at work.

I would get up early and work. I'd make the kids breakfast, get them off to school, come home and work. After school, I'd feed them, do mommy stuff, put them to bed, and then work some more.

This was not a happy time.

I began to go for short runs as a break from work. I'd listen to the cheesiest YA books about wizards or magical beings or werewolves while I ran. (I can recommend a few if you're interested.)

I allowed myself to run as slow as I wanted, stop whenever I felt like it, and each time I laced up my shoes I told myself, "I'm going running because I want to. Not because someone is telling me to."

I didn't run far, and I didn't run fast. But it became a source of refuge and release for me. I felt grateful for my legs that they could carry me. Grateful for the sky that it was so much bigger and more open than my office. Grateful for the birds that cheered me on as I ran. Grateful for the opportunity to stop and walk any time I wanted to. My runs became a gift I could give myself.

What if you were to shift your perspective on exercise away from viewing it as a punishment and toward viewing it as a gift to yourself?

Ex: *"I GET TO do this zumba class because it's fun, it is a stress reliever, and I like the way it feels to move my body. This is my gift to myself."*

Sometimes it helps to pair up exercise with something else that you already enjoy. For example, you could listen to a great book while you walk or watch Netflix while you exercise.

By coupling something you enjoy (the book, music, or Netflix) with something you feel like you should do (the exercise), you're associating good feelings with the movement.

What ways might you view exercise (any kind you like!) as a gift to yourself?

CHAPTER 11
HOW TO BE
MORE PRESENT

B ack when my husband and I first started dating, I had a relatively long commute to work. So instead of surfing channels
on the radio to find a good song, I just merrily tuned out whatever
music was playing and daydreamed about my honey.

I'd get so lost in my thoughts, that sometimes I'd look up and
be like "Wait. Where AM I? Oh yeah, my exit is two stops away."
Then I'd happily return to my gooey eyed musings and proceed
to miss my exit, making my commute even longer. "Aw man! I
did it again!"

Life is a Highway

We do this all the time with food. Your body is the highway, where
road signs are like subtle signals and sensations your body sends
you when you're eating. But you're so busy thinking about the
deadline for the TPS project at work or worrying about whether
Sally got your text and *"She hasn't messaged me back yet. Is she mad*

at me? Maybe I should text her again…" and suddenly you missed the exit that said, *"Hey, we're full. It's time to stop eating."*

You didn't even notice that signal from your body and you kept on trucking by. Now you've had way more food than you planned, with some guilt to go along with it. On top of that, now your bag of chips is empty. Sigh.

How do you learn to refocus your attention on the road signs and signals your body is sending you when your brain is yammering all the time?

One way is to put a number on it.

The Hunger Number

Imagine a number line with zero in the middle and +10 on one end and -10 on the other end. -10 is how you feel when you're famished or so hungry you could eat a house. +10 is how you feel when you ate way too much pizza and you need to put on your stretchy pants. Naturally, zero is neutral in the middle. It's how you feel when you're neither hungry nor full.

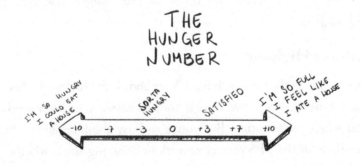

The Hunger Number gives you a numerical value to measure on how you feel at any given moment.

What you're aiming for is to never get below -3 or -4 and never get above +3 or +4. You want to eat when you feel a little bit hungry, and you want to stop eating when you feel a little bit full.

Have you ever skipped a meal, but then when you did decide to eat, it was hard to stop eating? That happens because when you get past -4 on the hunger scale, your brain goes into scarcity mode.

Your primitive brain wants to avoid starvation in case there is a famine. So when you do decide to eat, the subconscious signal from the brain is *"Eat as much as we can while there's still food available because we don't know when we'll get to eat again!"*

In addition, that healthy meal you planned no longer looks so good when you're past -4. The brain wants energy, stat! And it knows that certain kinds of foods have more energy (ie. calories) than others. You guessed it. Foods high in sugar, salt, and fat. So just notice when you're feeling hungry past -4 so you don't overcompensate when you do end up eating.

On the other end of the scale, stopping at or before +4 allows you to feel satisfied but not too full.

My dad always told me, *"Leave the party while you're still having fun because when you stay too long, it can ruin a good time."*

Eating to +3 or +4 is like that. You can wake up feeling ready for food the next day rather than trying to promise yourself that you'll only eat salad for the rest of your life because you feel so full.

The Hunger Number helps you to be in tune with your body. If you're eating chips out of the bag on the couch while watching Hulu, you're not so likely to be thinking about how your body feels. The Hunger Number reminds you to tune in every now and then and eat in a manner that feels good to your body, rather than just feeding your emotions.

A small way to start out using the Hunger Number can be simply to keep a record of how you feel on the number line at various times of day. Set a reminder in your phone to check in and gauge what number you'd give your hunger level every few hours. That can be a mini step in the direction of using the Hunger Number to help you determine when to eat and when to stop eating.

Eating In the Fast Lane

I'll be honest. When I first started thinking about mindful eating, I hated it. It felt more like "guilt-ful eating" than anything else. I like to Get. Stuff. DONE. Multitasking while I eat seems like a great way to kill two birds with one stone.

However, that's like eating in the fast lane of life.

When I do that, I can eat a whole meal and realize I never really tasted any of it. And it's MUCH easier to overeat when I'm not paying attention. Since I really love food, and I enjoy actually tasting it, and I don't love the feeling of being over-full, I learned to give mindful eating a fair shot.

For those who say that food is just fuel, good for them. But that alone ignores a whole host of other reasons why we eat.

We also eat because food is amazing! It tastes, smells, and feels so good! Food can be a way to express love. Food can be a beautiful form of communion with others. Combining food and time and conversation with others becomes so much more together than any of those elements are on their own.

Food is gorgeous and glorious and one of the most exquisite experiences of this life. Why oh why would we want to rush through that and miss it because we're looking at our phone?

Actually, a lot of reasons.

I love Friday night movie night with the family. I am not as focused on my food when we eat in front of the TV. But I accept the trade off because I enjoy the ritual.

Other times, I do take the time to stop and look at my food, smell it, thank God for the sunshine that helped grow it, and the people who helped it get to my plate. When we can be mindful and present with our food, we get so much more out of the experience.

Eating mindlessly can feel good in the moment. It's a way to numb, tune out, buffer, and ignore the emotions that you're feeling. While that has short-term pleasure, it has long term consequences. Both because the feelings you're numbing don't go away and the food you're shoveling is accumulating in unattractive ways. And you're not even actually tasting it!

Why eat mindfully?

- You actually get to enjoy the food you're eating.
- You are more likely to be able to tell when you're full.

- You get to be the one in charge of the decisions rather than reacting to the food or circumstances in your environment.

Frankly, there are times when I'm still not that great at mindful eating. But there are some easy ways to sneak in a little bit of mindfulness here and there to have your multitasking and taste your food too.

Here are some ideas to start experimenting with mindful eating.

Pick and choose or combine different ones. See what you like and what you don't. Customize what works for you.

- Try eating one meal a week or per day without a screen or any other distraction.
- Try pausing before eating and appreciating the colors of your food. The smell. The texture.
- If you're spiritually inclined, take a moment to thank God or the Universe for all that went into creating the food that you are blessed to eat and ask that it may nurture your body just as God nurtures your soul.
- Try putting your fork down between bites or after every third bite. Make it a game.
- Chew your food more. Take extra time to really chew it and taste it in your mouth.
- Stop eating after five minutes and wait two minutes before eating again. Check in with your body. How do you feel? What's been your favorite part of the meal so far? Do you want more or are you full?

- Slow down. Time yourself eating. Tomorrow, try and make the same meal take two minutes longer.
- As you're eating, try and label the sensations you're experiencing in your mouth and in your body. Name it. What does it taste like? Smell like? Etc.
- Make a deal with yourself that you can have any snack you want as long as it's at the table. Distraction free. Just you and the food.
- Sometimes when I'm trying to remember something, I move a ring to a different finger or a bracelet my daughter made me to the other wrist. It feels weird because it's not in the normal place.
  - It makes me be more present with myself and say, "Wait. Why is this on the wrong finger? What was I trying to remind myself of?"
  - That could be a way to help you remember to check in with yourself and ask if you're hungry or remind yourself to be present with your food.

There's no way to be perfect at mindful eating. (Perfection is not a thing!) There is no "right." It's just a question of do you want to enjoy the gift of food one percent more this week than last week? Treat it lightly. See what happens. Have fun with it.

Back Seat Driving

I used to really love pizza. I could easily eat four slices of pizza without hardly taking a breath. The smell of it alone was enough to ruin my diet.

The crazy thing was, it almost felt like I wasn't the one in control of making the choice to eat another slice. It was as if the back seat driver in my brain took over the wheel and said, *"I'm in charge here!"* However, that reactive eating left me feeling really bloated, painfully full, and all-around gross after eating pizza.

One morning after a particularly big night of pizza, I distinctly remember telling my husband, *"I think I want to break up with pizza."* He raised an eyebrow as if to say, *"Good luck with that."*

The conscious mind is where you decide, *"I'll just have one slice of pizza and a side salad."* Yet the subconscious mind is the one that takes over and says *"Screw the salad. I'll have three more slices and a side of bread sticks!"*

So which part of your brain gets to decide what to eat in the moment and how do you give your conscious mind a fighting chance when the subconscious mind is using weapons of diet destruction?

There are a couple of ways to give your conscious mind an edge.

Step 1: Be Aware Of Environmental Triggers
Sometimes the best laid plan can get wrecked simply by what's around us. Here are some of the things that can make you change your mind about what you decide to eat, no matter what your conscious mind said earlier in the day.

1) The presence of food.

    Simply by being present, a food can make you change your mind. Ever walked by the candy bowl in the office and randomly grabbed one on your way to the copier? Or maybe you hadn't had a thought in your mind about chips, but then your partner brought some home and now they're just THERE.

STARING AT YOU.

Be prepared for this in advance. Think ahead. What sort of food will be available? If you're going out, you know the breadbasket will be there. How do you want to respond to it in the moment?

In my case with the pizza, I knew I had to eat my side salad first, or it would never happen. That helped me get in some good greens first and feel fuller before starting in on the pizza.

2) What other people are eating.

Have you ever watched a commercial for something and thought, "Mmm, that looks good."

Watching other people eat triggers our mirror neurons. We are neurologically wired to mimic others in order to fit in with the tribe. So by seeing someone eat something, the mirror neurons light up the same areas of the brain that would fire if you had actually eaten the food. But since you didn't actually eat it, you now crave it.

So if you see someone eating dessert, be aware that your mirror neurons will tell you, *"I want some too."* It's not that you have faulty willpower. It's simply your brain doing what it does, thinking that it's helping you survive by fitting in with the tribe.

Knowing in advance can help you be prepared for that thought to come along and counter it with a proactive thought like, *"Yeah, I know that looks good, but it's not on my plan today. Maybe tomorrow."*

Have you ever changed your mind about what you plan to order at a restaurant based on what other people in the group ordered?

Again, our brains are wired to help us fit in with the tribe. Our survival literally depends on it (at least that's what the subconscious mind thinks.) So when you're the last one to order, you can be strongly influenced by what others ordered in front of you.

You can counter that by ordering first, or by reminding yourself that your survival does not actually depend on you ordering the same burger and cheese fries as the person at your table who ordered before you.

At the end of the day, it's not about other people. They don't really care about what you're doing. It's more about how it reflects on them. When you're in a place where you are confident in what you're doing, it really doesn't matter what other people are doing or thinking.

All the power is within you, and managing your own desire is within you. You don't have to control the external environment in order to change what you feel on the inside.

Step 2: Be Aware Of Emotional Triggers

There are so many reasons why we eat. And emotions account for about 4,739 of them. You already know that you're more likely to have less willpower later in the day because of decision fatigue and your brain has less resources available to make decisions that support long-term goals.

But whatever emotions are at play can accelerate that process. From the minor to the mighty, all kinds of ups and downs in your emotions throughout the day can impact your decisions around food later on.

Here are just a few examples:

- Logistics: *"Okay, Hannah has a soccer game this afternoon, but I have a work meeting at 2:30. I think I can make it on time if we wrap up when we're supposed to. But Roger is running the meeting and he's terrible about respecting other people's time. Oh, and it's my turn to bring the snacks, so I have to remember to stop by the store on the way. Ugh, Sarah brought homemade parfait fruit cups last week. She's like the perfect mom. My store-bought Cheetos and juice boxes are lame."* Etc.

- Boredom: *"I've been working on this report for two hours. It's time for a break. I know, how about a snack!"*

- Frustration: *"Why does my child refuse to put on his shoes exactly two minutes before we have to get out the door? Every. Damn. Time."*

- Worry / Anxiety: *"Why hasn't Amanda texted me back? Is she angry with me? I meant it as a joke. I hope she took it that way. Should I text her again and explain? Maybe I should say something. Maybe I should leave it alone. Maybe her phone fell in the toilet. I don't know!"*

- Grief: *"Mom's test results came back. They're not good."*

273

We are emotional beings that have thoughts. Not the other way around.

Just know that even something that seems small can create a cascade of emotions that drain your willpower and leave you vulnerable to the easy decision in the moment that doesn't serve you in the long run.

Step 3: Take Your Brain To The Gym

When you know there are certain foods that your brain wants, but your body feels bloated or tired afterward, you can train your brain to focus on different aspects that help you be in control of your choices.

Mentally, how can you strongly attach the bloated, tired feeling to that food that you'd like to have less of?

Whenever you have a craving for a food, there are two ways to look at it:

1) *"I want this food because I'm craving it at this moment, and I don't care about the consequences."*

2) *"I know this food will make my body feel gross later. How badly do I want to eat it knowing that I'll feel gross?"*

Just taking a pause and considering the option is a win! Even if you still decide to go for the not-so-healthy food. It's a win because you are putting yourself in control of your choices rather than reacting in the moment.

But you can take it a step further. Just like you're not gonna get stronger muscles by sitting on the couch, your thoughts aren't gonna change if you don't direct them on purpose.

- Proactively carve out time to think about how good healthy food makes you feel.
  - Attach your proactive thought time to something you already do regularly.
  - Ex: *"Okay, I am specifically trying to eat less bread. When I brush my teeth, I'll spend one minute proactively thinking about how great I feel when I eat healthy food and how gross I feel when I eat bread."*
- Take time to associate good feelings with healthy food.
  - If you're trying to avoid bread, proactively take a moment when you chose a meal without bread to give yourself a mental high five. Like *"Dang, I feel good! Whohoo! Go me!"* (Yeah, it's cheesy. Roll with it, my friend. You gotta be your own biggest cheerleader.)

It took me six years to get to the point of mindfully being aware of my pizza cravings, tasting the pizza as I ate it, noticing how my body felt afterwards and finally getting to a place where I legitimately would prefer a salad instead of a pizza slice.

Be patient. Give yourself the grace to feel like it's not working. It is. It just takes time.

Do I still have pizza? On occasion. But it doesn't pull at me the way it used to because I don't want the bloated, painfully full, gross feeling that I know comes with it.

There are still other foods like that for me that I'm working through the question of, *"Is the way I'll feel after I eat or drink this worth the feeling I get from it now?"*

Sometimes the answer is no, and I choose something else. Sometimes the answer is still yes, and I take the consequence of how I'll feel later as part of the bargain.

We're all a work in progress and that's ok.

PART 2
THE IMPERFECT TOOLBOX

Strategies and Tactics for Losing Weight In Real Life

What is an Imperfect Toolbox?

Listen, life is messy.

This whole book has been about how when we strive to be perfect, we fall flat. So let's make a plan for being imperfect. Let's embrace it! Perfection is boring anyway (if it were actually a thing.)

Weight loss is not about following the perfect plan. There is no perfect plan.

Nor is there such a thing as following a plan perfectly.

Life will present you with different circumstances on different days. When every day is different, you need a variety of tools to help you navigate the wild waters of weight loss.

Instead of giving you a plan to follow, I want you to have strategies that you can use to adjust to whatever situation life throws at you.

Think about the following section like filling your weight loss toolbox with a collection of strategies, tools, and tactics that you can draw from when you need them in different circumstances.

When life is real rather than perfect.

The following tools are meant to give you a path forward for specific weight loss challenges. I'm talking about things like weekends, holidays, snacking, etc. Not the latest 30 day challenge that will only entrench the diet mentality.

Try each one with curiosity. Treat it lightly. Have fun with it!

If something works, great!

If something doesn't work, great!

Remember, everything is like an experiment. All results are positive results because they are helping you learn more about yourself.

Weight loss is a skill.

Like any other skill, it takes a process of:

1. Try something
2. Mess up
3. Reflect
4. Learn
5. Repeat.

You've learned lots of skills in your life. You can learn the skill of weight loss too.

TOOL #1
How To Meal Plan

If you asked me, "What is the ONE, single most effective weight loss tool?" it would be meal planning.

Meal planning is a domino habit that makes everything else so much easier.

Real quick, I want to distinguish the difference between meal planning and meal prep.

Meal planning is simply sitting down and deciding what you'll eat in the next 24 hours or what meal(s) you will have on what days this week. You don't actually have to prepare the food you're planning in that moment.

Meal prep is often referred to as "batch cooking" where you make many servings of a single meal and portion it out and save it for lunches or various meals throughout the week.

Both tactics can be valuable.

Sometimes folks get caught up (and then discouraged) with meal prep because (a) it takes a while to cook and portion out all that food and (b) it can get boring to eat the same thing over and over again throughout the week.

If that's you, it's all good! Don't let that discourage you from at least doing a little meal planning.

First of all, why plan your meals?

- It takes away the decision fatigue of trying to figure out what to eat in the moment when you are often tired or stressed.
- You can make your plan when you are feeling more rested, have more willpower, and can make better decisions for yourself.
- Often you can also look ahead and predict what days that will be a little more hectic and plan a meal that is easy to cook and takes less time and less effort. *(Ex: "Johnny has basketball practice on Tuesday night. We won't get home until 7:15, so I'll need to plan for something quick and easy.")*
- You actually SAVE MONEY by not buying food you end up wasting because you don't eat it and not spending extra money on last minute take-out. Who doesn't like more dollars in their wallet?

Here are some common objections to meal planning:

- I don't have time.
  - Meal planning actually saves time in the long run.
- What if I don't feel like eating what I planned for that night?
  - No problem. Have a back-up plan or be willing to be flexible.
- I'm just too tired.
  - Planning reduces stress and fatigue because you're limiting the number of decisions you have to make. Incidentally, this also improves willpower because the less decisions you make, the less drain on willpower.

STRATEGIES AND TACTICS FOR LOSING WEIGHT IN REAL LIFE

- I don't know what to plan.
  - Make a list or a chart of five to seven meals the family likes and rotate them.

How To Get Started

There are lots of different ways to meal plan. You can (and should!) absolutely test, experiment, tweak and adjust the process to fit your life and your preferences.

Are you the kind of person who:

- Likes a little flexibility and be able to cook / eat "what you're in the mood for tonight?"
- Or do you prefer to know "X is for dinner tonight" so that you don't have to think about it?

Depending on the kind of person you are, you might resonate with one of the methods below:

- Flexible planning
- Fewer decisions panning
- One day at a time planning

1) Flexible Planning

If you're more of the kind of person who likes to feel what you're in the mood for, try an approach like this:

1) At the beginning of the week, identify four or five meals you'd like to have sometime this week.
2) Buy the ingredients for those meals.
3) Then when it comes time to cook, you know you can either have meal A, meal B, meal C, etc. You have a choice, with healthy boundaries.

That gives you a way to plan healthy meals for yourself while still giving you some wiggle room to flex in the moment.

2) Fewer Decisions Planning

If you like the idea of not having to think about it, try this:

Map out five to eight meals that you know you and the family enjoy. Then, plan out which meals you'll have on which nights of the week.

Plus, if you save your menus for the week, after a few weeks, you've got a treasure trove of plans so you don't have to keep reinventing the meal plan wheel.

For example:

- Monday is taco night. (Wait, shouldn't tacos be on Tuesday?)
- Tuesday is chicken with rice.
- Wednesday, I know I'll have to work late. So we'll plan to have a healthy take-out night at Panera or Moes.
- Thursday is turkey burgers with oven fries but no bun.
- Friday is steak with a side of broccoli.

Obviously, that's just an example.

But if you can identify meals you like and then plan ahead, that removes decision fatigue, and you end up saving time, money, and calories.

3) Just One Day At A Time Planning

If that's a little much for you, it's okay. Let's look at simply planning for one day at a time and making sure that the plan feels doable for you.

Here's how it works:

Each day, either the night before or the morning of, make a plan for what you want to eat during the day.

However, you have to put stuff on the plan that you ACTU-ALLY THINK YOU WILL WANT TO EAT.

That means if you think you'll want ice cream, put it on the plan.

If you think you'll want to graze on snacks, put it on the plan.

There is no food that is off limits.

The only rule is that if you have a craving for something that is not on your plan, you still get to have it.....tomorrow. When you've planned for it.

Give yourself the freedom to make a plan that you actually think you can stick to. Even if you think "I'll never lose weight eating this." That's okay!

You're creating the practice of showing up for yourself and following through on the promises you make to yourself.

Over time, if you want to start adjusting what goes on the plan, great. But ONLY if you think you will want to stick to it.

This is not about losing weight...YET. That will come in time.

This is about practicing the skill of learning to trust yourself and trust that you will only make promises to yourself that you know you will keep.

If you're thinking, *"The food I planned isn't good enough or healthy enough"* then you're doing it right. Because if you wanted to eat the way that the diet guru told you to, then you'd already be doing it.

Eat in a way that you can show up for yourself. Stop trying to be perfect and be honest with yourself about what you will ACTUALLY eat.

When you feel safe around food, you don't need to overcorrect with a binge because you're not depriving yourself. There's no making up for it the next day or needing to take a break over the weekend because you LIKE the way you're eating!

When you deprive yourself all week long, the problem is not the weekend. It's the restriction.

Decide that you are worth the time and thought it takes to plan out your meals.

Decide that you are worthy of telling yourself the truth about what you'll eat. You're always learning and that's okay! Make plans that are so easy they'll be hard to break.

You might be surprised that planning to have a treat food during the day actually results in eating less because you never get to the point where you think, *"Well, I screwed up the day so I might as well have more."*

If you decide to try this method, you might find yourself feeling guilty about how much overeating you've been doing.

Please hear this:

You've gotta drop the guilt.

Your past-self did the best she could. Please stop bullying your past-self. If you don't learn how to change the conversation with yourself then you will never learn to lose the weight and keep it off. If you are harsh and terrible to yourself, you will always be looking for diets that treat you in the same way.

You deserve better.

Start building TRUST with yourself.

No more punishing yourself for being overweight. You did nothing wrong. You just never got the opportunity to learn how to talk to yourself in a supportive way. It's time for that cycle to change. It is time for that mindset to change.

When To Plan

A great way to start with meal planning is first, to look at the calendar and pick a time of the week that you know you'll feel a little more rested and have the mental bandwidth to think out what you'd like to eat in the coming week. Weekends tend to work well, but again, adjust according to your life.

Then put it in your calendar. Make an appointment with yourself. If you need to, ask a friend to hold you accountable to actually doing it.

Next, figure out how many meals you want to plan. I usually start with dinners. That is the time of day that I am least on my game and most likely to say, *"Screw it. I don't feel like cooking."*

I don't especially love cooking. And I really don't love figuring out what's for dinner. So I do myself a favor by planning ahead so that I only have to think about it once during the week, rather than seven times a week.

Because I care about my future self and I know that I don't like thinking after 5 p.m., I give myself the gift of not having to think about what's for dinner except for just once a week. (I usually plan on Sunday mornings.)

Then look at the schedule. When is baseball practice? When are piano lessons? When do you have a work meeting that might go late? Think about what time you'll get home and plan accordingly.

How much time will you have to cook each evening? On nights when you have more time, you can plan for something that requires a little more attention. On nights when you're pressed for time, plan something super easy or quick.

Make It Easy

When you know you'll have less time to cook, make it easier to choose a healthy meal.

- Many stores have pre-cooked dishes or pre-cooked meat. All you have to do is pop it in the oven and bake for 25 minutes.
- There are plenty of in-the-bag microwavable veggies that are easy to prepare. Match up a protein and a veggie and you're done.
- Some nights are just made for take-out. Think ahead of the take-out places you like. What's the healthiest meal you can order there?

The idea is to give your future self a break by giving yourself the gift of not having to decide in the moment.

Meal Prep

If you decide that you want to do some food prep as well as meal planning, here are some ideas to get your started.

LUNCH:

Consider preparing a big batch of salad for the week. Then on a given day you can warm up a protein (pre-cooked chicken or last night's leftovers), portion out a serving of salad, top it with extras like hard-boiled egg slices, avocado, shredded cheese, and you're good to go. (Tip: I like salsa as a salad dressing because it's tasty and has few calories and very little sugar. Experiment with what works for you.)

SNACKS:

Try using weekend time to cut up a bunch of veggies. I like cut peppers and cucumbers, but carrots, broccoli, and cauliflower can work well too. Often there are pre-cut bags of veggies that are easy to grab at the store.

Generally speaking, if healthy food isn't easy to grab, then you're not likely to choose it. So once you pre-cut the veggies, bag them into single serving bags to make it as easy as possible to choose the healthy option during a busy day.

FOR THE KIDS:

If you have kids, there are lots of things they can help with to prep their lunches for the week.

Kids can bag up five days' worth of lunches that will go in their lunch bags each morning.

Pre-cut carrots and broccoli can be easy for kids to portion into bags for lunch. Five bags of each item for five days. On any given morning, all you have to do is grab one bag of pretzels, one bag of apples, one bag of cheese slices, one bag of veggies, toss it in their lunchbox and you're good to go!

- Usually people have more time on weekends. That can be a time to shop and batch prep stuff.

- If you know what the kids' lunches will be each day, grab the family and sort it out by day.
  - Ex: One kid is in charge of putting all the cheese slices into ziplock baggies.
  - One kid can be in charge of putting a handful of goldfish into baggies and counting out five for the week.
- If something requires cutting (like apples) you can be in charge of cutting and then have a kiddo place them in baggies.
- Rinse and repeat for each food item that goes in their lunch.

This ONE habit has made my mornings infinitely better. (Plus, now the kids are old enough to do it for themselves. SOOO GLORIOUS!) Give it a try!

Pre-Logging

If you've decided that you want to use an app to log your food and calories, sometimes it can be tedious to remember to log all your meals.

One thing that some people find helpful is to pre-log the foods and drinks they plan to eat during the day to check and see where that will put them in terms of total calories for the day.

This helps in two ways:

a) It gives you an idea of where you are in your budget and how much is too much. #awarenessforthewin!

b) It can serve as a pre-commitment device. It helps you make a small promise to yourself that "This is what I plan to eat." And even if you go off it a little, it's still better than no plan at all.

Alternative Ways To Food Log

Food logging is not for everyone. It's a great way to be more aware of the food you're taking in. But it can be tiresome, and it can lead to feeling a little obsessive about calories. Also, calorie counting can backfire. If you get discouraged early in the day, it can lead to giving up. Naturally, that's not going to lead to success.

In the long run, the goal is not to get really good at estimating how many calories are in a bowl of granola or in a serving of chicken cacciatore.

The goal is to get in touch with your body and learn what makes your body feel good while not getting overly full or excessively hungry.

Here are some other ways to be aware of and cognizant of what you're eating, while not obsessing over calories.

- Keep a pen and paper journal of what you eat during the day with a rough estimate of your portion size. No measuring. No calorie counting. Just what you ate.
- Do something similar but with a note on your phone, since your phone is likely to be with you when your piece of paper or journal may not.
- Keep a photographic log of what you eat. If it goes in your mouth, take a picture of it. That way you don't have to write things down, but you have a record that you can refer to so you know what you ate.

All of this is simply data. The data is helping you and informing you along your journey.

If the scale goes up, you can look back at your food log (again, not calorie counting) and see what might be contributing to that.

The bigger goal is to help you begin to tune into your body's signals and learn what feels good, what feels too full, what makes you feel sluggish, or makes you sleep poorly, etc.

These are all data points that you can use to learn over time how to eat in a way that serves you rather than restricts you.

TOOL #2
How To Experiment with Intermittent Fasting

There is a lot of research out there about intermittent fasting (I.F.) and how it can be a healthy lifestyle. There was a time in my life when I thought there was no way I would EVER want to try intermittent fasting. I love breakfast food and the whole idea sounded miserable to me.

However, like so many things, that was just a thought. A sentence in my brain that was only true if I decided it was true. So I began to ask myself some questions.

- Do I *have* to have breakfast every day?
- How does my body feel when I'm eating food for most of the day?
- What if I experimented with something different?

While I.F. may not be for everyone, I found it to be a useful experiment for me and it can be something to experiment with if you want to try it.

Here's why it works:

The body will always use sugar (or carbs) as an energy source before fat because fat is like the storage vault of energy that it wants to save for a rainy day. Or a famine.

It's like a bank account.

- Carbs are the checking account.
  - They're easy fuel and the body will draw from that first.
- Protein is the savings account.
  - The body will draw from protein as a fuel source after carbohydrates.
- Fat is the retirement account.
  - Money you put in a retirement account is income you're saving for "later." Fat is the same way in the body. The body wants to save fat as a fuel source because it stores more energy. So in a way it's more "valuable" to the body as a last resort. The body is really good at keeping you alive so it wants to save all the fat it can in case it needs to draw on that energy "someday."

When you sleep through the night, the body is burning through your carb and protein fuel sources because you're not introducing any new fuel into the body during that time.

After roughly twelve hours, the body has usually burned up the available carb and protein stores so that's when it starts to go to the fat reserves.

If you stopped eating early the night before, then there's a longer window of time where there's no new fuel coming into the body overnight. This gives your body more time to draw from those fat stores.

On the other hand, if you eat late, by the time you get up in the morning, the body may not have had enough time to get to the fat burning mode. If you add in new fuel in the morning, then it never needs to turn to fat as a source of fuel.

When I first tried intermittent fasting, I decided to just do it on Sundays. That was not a good plan because I usually had less going on to keep me busy on those days. So I was thinking about food A LOT.

Then I tried just Tuesdays and Thursdays. That was better because I was busy during the mornings. However, I'd wake up and feel deprived like *"Oh. Today is a fasting day. I guess I don't get to eat breakfast today."*

That feeling of deprivation can accumulate over time and it's not helpful. When I decided to try fasting every day and just make it "my new normal," that made everything SO much easier! I still have breakfast on occasion, but it is more the exception than the rule.

As with everything, experiment with what works for you. Tweak it along the way and listen to yourself. Your body has wisdom.

Typical methods for I.F. include 16:8 or 18:6. That means 16 or 18 hours of fasting and a window of 8 to 6 hours of eating.

When you break the fast, it's a good idea to take it slow. Eat normally or start with a small snack. Also, whatever you eat will hit your blood stream faster because you don't have anything in your stomach already. Therefore, you want to avoid sugary or starchy foods as the first thing you eat because that will spike your blood sugar. Smoothies can seem like a great idea, but they often have lots of sugar, so they may be better at the end of a meal or as a snack.

TOOL #3

How To Make Weekends
Your Weight Loss Friend

Why is it that we can be "good" all week and then we blow all our progress on the weekends and start over again on Monday right in the same place where we started a week before (or worse)?

It can seem unfair that five days' worth of hard work can be undone in just two days of less structured eating. You may find yourself wondering *"Will I ever be able to just relax on the weekend again and not worry about what I eat?"*

It's understandable to want a break on the weekends. Our work life slows down on weekends, so it's natural to want that to apply to what we eat as well.

However, if the way you eat during the week is something that you feel like you need a break from or need to "cheat," then it's not going to be sustainable long term.

Imagine the way you eat is like a life partner.

How would your life partner feel if you said, *"I love you Sunday-Friday, but Saturdays I'm gonna see other people."*

You want to find a life partner that you WANT to spend all seven days of the week, 365 days of the year with.

It's the same with your eating lifestyle. Sure, variety is fine. But you want to eat in a way that you don't need to cheat or stray from it because you actually LIKE the way you normally eat.

If you think about it, the weekend often starts on Friday night. So the weekend ends up being about 35% of the entire week.

If you're off target 35% of the time, that can really add up.

How might your behavior change if you went into the weekend planning to lose weight by Monday?

Let's start with the end in mind.

How do you want to feel on Monday morning? Bloated, regretful, and starting over? Or do you want to feel like you were in control of your choices?.

Once you decide how you want to feel on Monday, then reverse engineer your plans and your mindset over the weekend to make that Monday vision a reality.

At the end of the day, the goal is to create a lifestyle that you don't need a break from on weekends.

Practically speaking, set aside some time on Thursday night to look ahead to your weekend. I know some people that meal plan twice a week. Once on Sunday for Monday-Thursday and then again on Thursday for the weekends because you don't always know what the weekend plan will be on the Sunday prior.

So on Thursday night, map out what your weekend plans are. Then strategize your meals around that. What will you have for breakfast if you sleep in? Will you be going out to a restaurant for dinner one night? If so, plan ahead (see below for restaurant info) and make a game plan for what you'll eat there. Do you plan to drink over the weekend? If so, how much would make you feel good? How much would be too much?

You may be thinking, "There's no way my family will go for that. Plus, I like to have a little flexibility and spontaneity."

No worries.

What if you set up SYSTEMS for yourself rather than rules? For example:

- *"When I don't know what we're going to eat, I'll at least try and make sure there's a veggie or salad option available and eat that first to fill my stomach with healthier food."*

- *"When I don't know what we're going to eat, I'll know that I want to be even more mindful of portions. So I'll serve myself 1/4 less than what I think I might want to eat, knowing I can always have more."*

Too often we spend the whole weekend being reactive. Reactive to whatever happened during the week. Reactive to whatever plans happen to pop up. Reactive to our whims, emotions, and feelings in the moment.

Be proactive about your weekends and allow your planning brain to be in the driver's seat. Do you want to let life happen to you? Or do you want to plan to make life happen FOR you?

TOOL #4
How To Not Blow Everything When Eating at Restaurants

Eating out can be a danger zone. It's easy to overeat because the servings are large, and you're faced with having to make decisions in the moment. Spur of the moment decisions often are ones we end up regretting later.

There are a couple of ways to pre-manage a restaurant meal that you might explore.

1) A lot of restaurants have their nutritional info listed on their website.

   Just search "[restaurant name] nutrition info" and see if you find anything. If you do, then you can pre-plan your meals according to how many calories you'd like to "spend" on your meal out.

2) If they don't have their nutritional info listed, no problem. Look up their menu online and see what meals interest you.

   Then go to a meal logging app of your choice and pre-log a meal that is similar. You're not likely to find that exact meal, but you can often find things that are very close.

This will give you a ballpark idea of how many calories that dish likely has. Then you can make a more informed meal choice when you get to where you're going.

3) If you don't know where you're going ahead of time, you can always use strategy #2 once you get there.

However, if you don't want to get your phone out as you're deciding on your meal, a small salad as a starter will help you feel full sooner and help you guarantee to get some healthy food in.

Bonus Tips:

Remember how starchy carbs (like bread) and salty foods hold on to water in the body? Try to avoid the bread bowl or the chips and salsa either by asking the server not to bring it or place it far away from you on the table.

If you love chips and salsa, great! Portion some out on a plate. Identify how much you want to have and mentally tell yourself, "This is my serving of chips." Put as much on there as you want, but allow yourself to SEE it all at once. We get ourselves into trouble with the chips because just eating one at a time makes it easy to lose track of how much you've had.

Keep in mind that restaurants tend to add a lot of salt and butter to their cooking methods to make their food tastier. So if the scale is up the next day, try not to sweat it. It's likely water weight.

Also, be mindful of what you're thinking when at a restaurant. A lot of times we open the menu and think *"Look at all these things I can't eat."* That doesn't help. It makes you feel disempowered and whiny about being on "a diet."

Instead, open the menu and ask yourself "*What's the healthiest thing on this menu? What would make my body feel amazing tomorrow?*" If it turns out you don't want that, it's fine. Then look for the next healthiest thing. Start out with a positive frame of mind about how you want to show up versus telling yourself a lousy story about what you "can't" have.

TOOL #5
How To Manage Portions

Portion control can be a crazy thing. Our brains think we want more than our bodies actually need. However, if the food is just right there in front of you, it can be SO hard to not eat it, even if you know you're not hungry!

There's a great book called Mindless Eating[30] by Brian Wasnik that goes into deep detail about the science behind portion control.

For example, people will eat more popcorn if it's from a larger bag, even if it is old and stale. People also have poor judgment about how much they ate. When a soup bowl is designed to refill itself without the eater knowing, the eater will eat much more soup than just a normal serving.

We use our eyes to tell us how much we ate more than we use our body sensations. When food comes served on large plates or in big servings, our eyes are not the best judge of how much we ate.

<u>Bottom line</u>: We are really bad at knowing when we're full.

If you're in the early stages of practicing getting in tune with your body and being aware of fullness cues, also try using some portion control hacks (below) to help you along the way.

---

30 Mindless Eating by Brian Wasnik

The key is to plan ahead and think about how to hack your habits before the food is sitting in front of you.

First, you need to identify when you're more likely to eat an oversized portion. Common culprits include:

- Eating at restaurants
- Serving yourself for dinner
- Eating directly from a bag or box
- Serving yourself dessert

Here are some tips and tricks to make it easier to start small, knowing you can always go back for more.

- Always portion out food from a box or a bag onto a smaller serving dish. Put the box or bag away. Make it a lot of effort to have to get up and give yourself more.

- If you do decide to go for seconds, set a timer between portions. Allow yourself five or ten minutes before getting seconds. Often that pause gives your planning brain time to say *"Actually, I think I'm good for now."*

- Use smaller plates. Research shows the brain will think you ate more if it looks like it takes up more room on your plate.

- Use smaller utensils. You can put less food on a smaller fork, therefore that forces you to take more bites, making your brain feel like you ate more.

- Serve up the amount you normally would have for dinner or dessert, then put ¼ of it back. See if you're still hungry for it later.

- Don't have the serving dishes at the table. Make it harder to get more food by leaving it in the kitchen.

- Only eat at the table. If you're trying to snack less, make a deal with yourself that you can eat whatever you want but it has to be sitting at the table with no other distractions. Just you and the food.
- At restaurants, ask the server for a to-go box when they bring out your meal. Portion out half of it when it arrives. Or ask the server to portion half of it into the to-go box before it gets to the table, so you don't have to decide how much is half.
- If you feel full and there's still food on your plate, it's easy to keep picking at it if it's just there in front of you. Once you're done, place a napkin over the food you don't want to eat. This signals to both you and your server that you're finished.
- At fast food places, order the smaller sizes or even the kids' sizes and see if you're still hungry later.

TOOL #6

How To Reduce Sweets

While I've technically heard of people that don't like sweets, the concept feels a little foreign to me. For the rest of us mortals trying to eat less sugar, here are some strategies and tactics to explore.

Strategies:

These are more process-oriented goals that give you a method for addressing sweets. Choose one option to try at a time (not all four at once!)

NOTE: These strategies can work for afternoon or late-night snacking as well.

1) Work on trying to improve the quality of the sweet treats.
2) Try to have a smaller portion size of sugary stuff.
3) Plan for a sugar treat at a specific time of day so you're more present with it. Choose the food with your proactive mind rather than being reactive to the moment.
4) Or aim for a certain number of days with no snacking on sugary treats and see how you feel.

Tactics:

These are more action-oriented goals that give you a specific action to help you create balance with sweets.

• The order in which you eat your food MATTERS.

When you eat a meal, it's not just a collection of calories. The order that you eat various nutrients impacts your blood sugar which influences your cravings.

Whatever you put in your stomach first is what gets digested first. If you're having a turkey sandwich with lettuce and tomato, you'll actually experience fewer sugar cravings later if you disassemble the sandwich, eat the lettuce, then the tomato, then the turkey, and the bread last.

It's the same number of calories, but by having the lettuce first and then the tomato, you're giving your body a food that has a lower impact on blood sugar than the bread.

As a rule of thumb, eat your nutrients in this order:

- Vegetable (fiber)
- Protein (meats)
- Fat (cheese, etc)
- Starch (potatoes, bread, rice, etc)
- Sugar (dessert)

  For more info on this, check out The Glucose Revolution by Jessie Inchauspe.[31]

- Give yourself a challenge to only eat [X] many sweets in a day. Try and reduce that number over time.

- Have a glass of water before allowing yourself a treat. Check in with your body to see how hungry you are and how the water might impact your desire for the treat.

- Allow yourself a treat only after you've had a healthy snack first.

---

31 The Glucose Revolution by Jessie Inchauspe

- If there's a big batch of treats, freeze most of them. Then when you're ready for a treat, plan it out and thaw just a single portion size as a way to prevent you from eating all of them (or a lot of them) at once.

- Give yourself a cut off time. Like *"I can have a snack up till 9 p.m., then I'm done."*

- Try having a moderate amount and if you still want more give yourself a wait time (Ex: ten minutes) after which you'll re-check in with yourself and your body to see if you still want it.

- Make an agreement with yourself that you're allowed to have more of the sweet snack you want, but only after you journal all the thoughts and feelings in your head that might be increasing your cravings. This strategy can be very powerful.

- You can try allowing the craving by leaning into the feeling and welcoming it, but not acting on it. Just let it be there.

- Sometimes creating a plan ahead of time for your post-meal treat can be a good way to give your brain a reward to look forward to, but there are boundaries around it.

What's interesting is that some folks notice that after they reduce or eliminate sugar, it changes their taste for it.

There is a scientific reason for that.

The cells in your taste buds live for about ten days to two weeks. When you eat a lot of sugar, those taste buds develop a "high tolerance" for sugar, so sweets don't taste as sugary.

When you go off sugar for a while, those high tolerance taste buds die off and the new ones that replace them don't have the same high level of tolerance because they've not been introduced to as much sugar.

So over time, your taste for sugar changes.

Just a little nerdy science there for ya!

TOOL #7
How To Handle a Snack Attack

I used to look forward to my afternoon snack like it was a prize I'd won or a reward for making it that far in the day.

The kids would get home from school, and they were hungry. I'd set them up with something to eat. It looked pretty good, so I'd give myself some too. Then there were the days when I'd start to snack, and I just couldn't seem to stop. It was like once the seal was broken, my brain didn't have an off switch.

It didn't take long for me to eat so much that I had no appetite for dinner. But I'd eat it anyway because that's what I was *supposed* to do. I'd go to bed feeling gross and vow to start fresh tomorrow.

Having a plan for snacks can save you from the 3:37 p.m. snack attack and help you set yourself up for success.

The same strategies that work for sweets apply to snacks as well.

1. Plan a snack ahead of time for the time of day that you tend to feel hungry. Plan for something that you will enjoy and look forward to but maybe is slightly healthier than what you were eating before.

2. Make a plan for the portion size you want to eat. Decide ahead of time how much is an amount that would help

you feel satisfied and how much would you end up regretting later.

3. Plan a snack that you will enjoy (though ideally somewhat healthy) and aim to really be present with the food you're eating. Sit at the table with no distractions. Just you and the food. Make it worth it and savor it.

4. Try experimenting with a day or two in the week where you plan to skip a snack and see how you feel. Notice your thoughts that come up. How does your body feel? Be a scientist and collect data on yourself!

Sometimes after dinner snacking can be a real challenge. It's late. You're tired but not ready to go to bed. It's easy to find yourself walking back to the pantry for more when you're watching TV or possibly had a glass of wine.

Here are some ideas for minimizing the damage of late-night snacks:

- Ask someone in your home for help. Let them know what your goals are and see if they can become your supporter versus tempter. See how the two of you might work together.

- If you decide to have a snack, always portion it out on a plate or small bowl. Never eat directly from the bag or box.

- Decide before dinner how much of the evening snack you plan to have. Don't decide in the moment. Give yourself a non-food reward for sticking to your plan.

- Brush your teeth after dinner or after the snack you've planned for yourself. Let that be a signal to yourself that you're done eating.
- Create a nighttime routine. Give your brain a consistent signal that says, *"It's time to start winding down."* For example, have decaf tea and let that be your brain's signal that you're done eating. Or change into your sleep clothes and make that the mental demarcation line that it's time to stop eating and wind down for the night.

How To Avoid Junk Food When It's Already in The House

Birthdays, holidays, the in-laws come to visit...all of these can be reasons why you might find extra tempting food in your house that's not normally there. When that happens, here are some strategies to help you navigate the minefield and get back on track quickly.

1. Remove the junk food from the house. Simply throw it out. Otherwise, you're using your body as the trash can. Or you can bring it into the office. Have the kids take it to school. Donate it to the local fire station.

2. If that's not an option, try putting the food in a different place or ask your partner to put it somewhere that they can access but you don't know where it is, so that it's not tempting you all the time.

3. Freeze things that are freezable so that it forces you to choose a moderate portion by having to thaw it first.

4. Put more tempting food in an opaque box so that you can't readily see if by just walking by.

5. If you decide to have some of the treat, as always, portion it out on a plate or in a small bowl so that you're never eating straight from the bag or box.

TOOL #8
How To Handle Stress Eating

Stress eating can cause more stress because you end up feeling lousy about yourself in the end and that perpetuates the cloud of negative thinking about yourself and your body.

Let's look a little deeper. What does your brain REALLY want in that moment when stress or boredom have piled up?

Most likely it wants a nice little distraction from work or stress. Your brain is tired, and it wants a break. However, trying to say *"Every time I notice a craving, I'll go fold the laundry instead"* doesn't work.

Why not?

Because folding the laundry doesn't give your brain that hit of dopamine and serotonin. It's about the reward that your brain gets. (Though I do know some folks that feel great satisfaction in getting the laundry folded. So if that's you, go for it.)

When you want to stress eat, how can you challenge yourself to find something quick and fun to do instead of grabbing food? There are lots of ways you can give your brain what it's looking for without food.

Here are some ideas:
- Challenge yourself to text puppy pictures to three friends.
- Play five minutes of a game on your phone.
- Do a sudoku puzzle.

- Go sit outside for a few minutes and enjoy the sunshine. Look at a plant, and breathe non-recycled air.
- Read a fiction book for ten minutes. (But avoid the news or social media. There is lots of research indicating that news and social media make your brain feel worse in the long run.)

It's understandable that healthy eating goes out the window when you're stressed. Stress has a way of making us narrow our focus on the urgent thing at hand, while we also widen our focus on the amorphous "stuff" that we're worried about. Which means things like self-care take a back seat.

But let's look at it a different way. What if during times of stress, those self-care practices are even MORE important?

Sort of like a seat belt.

You can get away with not wearing your seat belt if you're just moving the car from one parking spot to another, but you really want to be wearing that sucker when you're on the interstate going 75 mph.

What if your proactive de-stressing, self-care practices are like seat belts? The busier and faster life gets, the more important they are.

(For more, please revisit the chapter on How To Stop Eating Your Feelings.)

TOOL #9
How To Handle Increased Cravings From Exercise

Sometimes when you're getting into exercise for the first time or ramping up your exercise routine and frequency, you might notice more cravings.

It makes sense that your body might be asking for more fuel since you're taxing it in a different way.

You can either be patient and allow your body to acclimate, which generally takes about two to four weeks. Or you can look for healthy ways to add in more healthy calories intentionally. If you choose option two, aim for quality protein sources. I'm personally a fan of mixing cottage cheese or unflavored Greek yogurt with some chocolate protein powder. You do you.

If you notice that you're specifically having sugar cravings, that's a little different. Most likely that's happening because your muscles are sore.

Pain drains your willpower.

As you know, when your willpower is low, your brain wants more energy fast. And it knows that sugar is a fast way to get cheap energy.

So the candy or chocolate cravings are more about being tired and sore and less about your body needing more fuel.

Be patient with yourself. Slightly elevated cravings are normal. Try not to overcompensate by adding in lots of extra calories.

Also, drink more water.

Water is really helpful for helping your muscles heal and grow as you stress them by lifting weights or moving more. If you're not drinking enough, that can make cravings higher.

<u>Note:</u>

If you are lifting weights, it's common to see the scale stand still or even move up a little. The microtears that lifting creates in the muscle need to be healed. The body creates inflammation as the first response when healing takes place. So there is a little extra fluid in your body as that soreness is working its way out.

Don't freak out about the scale. It's normal!

TOOL #10
How To Drink More Water (and Why)

One piece of advice you often hear to help you lose weight is to "Drink water." That's great, but does water REALLY help you lose weight?

Yes.

And here's why:

- Often what our brains interpret as hunger is actually thirst. The body can live without food but not water. So if you're low on water, the survival part of your brain knows that many foods have water in them and can serve to hydrate you. So if you drink water, you may find that the feeling of hunger goes away.

- Also, drinking water can fill up your stomach. If you have a full glass of water ten minutes before you eat, you'll feel full sooner. Thus eat less.

- Your cells are about seventy percent water. If you're dehydrated, there's less available energy in your cells. Of course that impacts your brain, meaning your decision making is compromised when you have less water in your system.

  o Less brain power equals poor decisions.

So drink your water!

And yet, sometimes that's easier said than done.

If you struggle to find ways to drink more water, try pairing up water with things they already do during the day.

For example:

- Water when you first wake up.
- Have water with meals or every time you eat.
- Drink water when you check email.
- Enjoy a glass of water after walking the dogs.
- Have a glass of water first thing when you get home from work, etc.

Some people wonder about putting flavors in their water. In my opinion, if something helps you drink more water, then go for it.

NOTE: Drinks with caffeine actually dehydrate you a little bit because caffeine is a diuretic. So if you're having coffee, caffeinated tea, or sodas, try and add a glass of water to go with it.

TOOL #11
How To Feel Good In Your Clothes

Most often when people tell me they want to lose weight, it is because they want to feel confident and comfortable in their clothes.

That's great!

However, what they mean is they want to feel great in the clothes that used to fit when their body was smaller. Buying bigger clothes can feel like giving up. It feels shameful and defeating to buy a pair of pants in a bigger size.

There's nothing wrong with wanting to look and feel great in clothes you used to wear! However, by wearing clothes that don't fit well, you're reminding yourself every minute of the day that you don't like the size of your body. When that happens, the typical reaction is to restrict yourself by saying "I can't have XYZ."

That drains willpower.

If you're forcing yourself to wear clothes that don't make you feel good, you're stirring up more negative thoughts. Because of the restriction, now you have less willpower to handle those painful thoughts in healthy ways.

You're effectively programming in default thoughts that demoralize you, shame you, and leave you with less willpower to make positive decisions throughout the day.

It's like throwing wood on the fire and adding gasoline and wondering why it burns so fast.

Negative thoughts breed negative feelings. Negative feelings lead to overeating and thinking "Screw it!" after one small misstep.

Listen, I get that you don't want to buy new clothes in a bigger size. But your body is the way it is today.

All you have is today anyway. Because tomorrow will soon be today.

In order to get to the body you want tomorrow, you've got to do what you can to feel good about yourself TODAY. And the only reason why you think you want that "body of tomorrow" is because of how you think it will make you FEEL....comfortable and confident in your clothes.

So why not choose to feel that way TODAY and give yourself the best shot at feeling comfortable and confident by wearing the clothes that fit your body now? Buy something that looks good and FEELS good, not tight and uncomfortable. Wear something that makes you feel awesome!

You deserve to feel good! Your body deserves to be clothed in garments that fit today. That will help you love yourself all the way down the scale toward the clothes that you love at a different size.

Why WAIT to feel good? Why push that feeling off until tomorrow? Tomorrow is perpetually out there and not here.

Don't wait until you lose weight to wear clothes that make you feel good. No matter what size you are, give yourself and your body the love and respect to open up to feeling confident and comfortable in your clothes TODAY.

Appreciating yourself and your body is allowing yourself to become who you always wanted to be.

Unabashedly.

TOOL #12

How To Not Get Wrapped Up in Your Thoughts

The following are specific tools developed by really smart people to help you take a tiny sidestep outside of the story you're telling yourself in your brain and look at it from a different point of view.

It's hard to read the label when you're inside the jar.

These tools help you step outside the jar of your own head and see your thoughts for what they are. Just a story you're telling yourself. From there you can decide if you want to keep that story or tweak it to something better that serves you.

Acceptance and Commitment Therapy

Acceptance and Commitment Therapy[32] was developed by clinical psychologist Steven C. Hayes to help himself through his own debilitating anxiety.

The idea behind this technique is to simply gain some distance between yourself and the thought creating anxiety or discomfort. Remember, just because you have a thought, does not mean it is true.

---

32 https://stevenchayes.com/

Step 1: Recognize and identify the thought. ("I want to eat the cake.")

Step 2: Insert these words in front of the thought: "**I'm having the thought that** [insert thought]."

Say this out loud two or three times.

- "I'm having the thought that I want to eat the cake."
- "I'm having the thought that I want to eat the cake."
- "I'm having the thought that I want to eat the cake."

Step 3: Insert these words in front of the thought: "**I notice** I'm having the thought that [insert thought].

Say this out loud two or three times.

- "I notice I'm having the thought that I want to eat the cake."
- "I notice I'm having the thought that I want to eat the cake."
- "I notice I'm having the thought that I want to eat the cake."

As you get more distance from the thought you can see that it's just a thought. Like a balloon on a string slowly floating away from you.

You may notice that there are often a number of thoughts that are related to this one thought.

For example:

"I want to eat cake. Every time I go by the bakery section in the grocery store, the cake is there and so are the cookies. It's so hard to resist! It's not fair. Plus we're going over to my parents' house tonight.

Mom always pushes food on me like pumpkin bread or something. It's so good but I can't have it." etc. etc.

Imagine that your mind is like an attic and there are lots of boxes in the attic. These thoughts that are all related to each other are like a tangled ball of string. If you could put all the tangled strings of related thoughts into one box, how would you label this box?

The next time you notice yourself having a thought related to something that causes anxiety, you can interrupt the pattern by thinking, *"Oh, I'm pulling out the box in my mind labeled 'I can't eat baked goods.' I notice I'm rummaging around in that old story again."*

That can help you gain a little distance from your thoughts. The more distance you get, the less you identify with the thought as totally and unequivocally true.

The Work

The Work[33] is a simple yet amazingly effective tool developed by Byron Katie. It utilizes straightforward questions to help you look at the story you're telling yourself from a different angle and see if there might be a different way of looking at things.

Just opening up your mind to ask yourself a question in a different way can ease a lot of self-created suffering.

In weight loss, we often struggle with the push / pull dynamic in our brains when we tell ourselves we want something that we can't have.

---

33 https://thework.com/

Let's take cake, for example. Imagine you're walking through the grocery store, and you walk past the bakery section. There in the center of the aisle on display is a type of cake that you enjoy.

The primitive part of your brain that is driven by desires wants the cake. And the more rational part of your brain says *"Nope. I can't have the cake because I'm on a diet."*

We create a lot of suffering for ourselves when we tell ourselves the story, *"It's not fair that I can't have X."*

Here's how you might use The Work to examine the story *"I want the cake but I can't have it."*

Part 1: 4 Questions

Question 1: Is it true?

Statement: *"I want the cake, but I can't have it."*

In that moment, as you walk through the grocery aisle, is it true that you want the cake? Is it true that you cannot have it?

=> Often the answer is yes, because it FEELS really true.

Question 2: Can you absolutely know it's true?

In that moment, as you walk through the grocery aisle, can you absolutely know it's true that you want the cake and you cannot have the cake?

=> Often this question puts a little crack in the story we're telling ourselves.

a) Do you actually, 100% want the cake? What part of you doesn't want the cake?

b) Can you actually have the cake if you want it? What is preventing you from having the cake?

<u>Question 3</u>: How do you react, what happens, when you think that thought?

How do you react, what happens, in that moment as you walk through the grocery aisle, when you believe the thought that you want the cake but you cannot have it?

==> All sorts of things can come up here. What do you realize here?

a) How do you treat yourself in that moment as you walk through the grocery aisle (in your thoughts and behaviors)?

Ex: *I treat myself very poorly. I add a lot of shame and guilt. I feel bad because I want something I can't have. And then I feel bad for wanting it.*

It's like a double dose of bad feelings.

b) How do you treat others in the situation (in your thoughts and behaviors)?

Ex: *I get grumpy, and I can take it out on my kids or my spouse when I get home from the store. I end up not wanting what I planned for dinner. Sometimes we change the plan to eat out and I end up overeating to compensate for the empty feeling of not having what I wanted earlier in the day.*

c) In that moment as you walk through the grocery aisle, how do you feel in your body when you think this thought?

Ex: *My shoulders feel tight and hunched. I feel a heaviness in my chest and almost a burning sensation in my stomach.*

<u>Question 4</u>: Who would you be without the thought?

Who would you be without the thought, *"I want the cake but I cannot have it"* in that moment as you walk through the grocery aisle?

=> Everything is the exact same, but you are not capable of having the thought *"I want the cake, but I cannot have it."*

What happens then?

> Ex: *I feel lighter. I am free of this cloud of judgment and wanting but not having. I can just go through the store and finish my shopping and feel fine.*
>
> *I probably am more likely to have a healthy dinner that night than go off plan and get take-out.*

Part 2: The Turnarounds

From there, we can get into some turnarounds. These are statements that look at the original thought from different angles to see where there might be some ways to relieve the suffering caused by the thought.

To the Opposite:

- Original statement:
  - ○ *"In that moment in the grocery aisle, I want the cake, but I can't have it."*
- Turnaround:
  - ○ *"In that moment in the grocery aisle, I don't want the cake."*
  - ○ Or *"In that moment in the grocery aisle, I can have the cake."*
- What are two or three examples of how the turnaround to the opposite might be true?

To the Other:

- Original statement:
  - *"In that moment in the grocery aisle, I want the cake, but I can't have it."*
- Turnaround:
  - *"The cake wants me, but it can't have me."*
- Even if it sounds a little nonsensical, what are two or three examples of how the turnaround to the other might be true?

To the Self:

(Often you can substitute in "my thinking" or "my thoughts" if turning it around to yourself doesn't immediately make sense.)

- Original statement:
  - *"In that moment in the grocery aisle, I want the cake, but I can't have it."*
- Turnaround:
  - *"My thinking wants the cake, but my thinking can't have it."*
- What are two or three examples of how the turnaround might be true?

The Work is a simple tool but not necessarily an easy one. Take some time to walk through this and write out your thoughts. See what happens.

Again, the main purpose of this is to simply gain some distance between you and the thought so that you no longer identify with it quite so tightly. It opens up some room to allow a different perspective and ease the suffering that the original thought is causing you.

Victim Drama Triangle

Sometimes we find ourselves overeating or numbing out with food because of the feelings that we don't want to feel. There are any number of feelings that can be painful based on the things we have experienced and the stories we tell ourselves about those experiences.

While I would never ever invalidate or question someone's lived experience (trauma is real), we can sometimes perpetuate the suffering we feel based on the meaning we make and the stories we create around the experience.

This can range from the truly traumatic to the more mundane.

One common story I hear more often from women is some version of *"I am so busy taking care of everyone else that I just don't have time to take care of myself."*

It makes sense that many of us have some version of this story in our heads.

Just like anything, we can take caring for others too far. When we neglect our needs in service of others, that can breed feelings of resentment, martyrdom, and anger.

When we do that, we find ourselves falling into the role of the victim in the Karpman Drama Triangle[34], developed by Dr. Stephen Karpman in 1968 to describe high-conflict situations.

The Karpman Drama Triangle, also called the victim triangle, describes the roles people play in the shifting dynamics of a conflict in a relationship.

---

34 https://www.karpmandramatriangle.com/

There are three roles in a conflict:
- Victim
- Persecutor
- Rescuer

The Victim

You're probably a busy person. We've all got a lot going on, and it's easy to feel overwhelmed sometimes by all the things we need to get done.

However, we put ourselves in the victim role when we allow ourselves to feel powerless to make decisions to change things or dependent on others or external circumstances.

Problems feel unsolvable, outside of our control, and it's easy to blame the perpetrator, which can be a situation, a person, or circumstance.

For example:
- *I have three kids and a full-time job. There's no time to meal plan and by the time dinner comes around I'm too tired to cook something healthy.*
- *My husband and kids don't like healthy food, and I don't want to cook two different meals for them and me.*
- *I'm always hungry after dinner. I just can't help it.*

When we allow ourselves to play the victim role, that feels bad! It's not a big leap to go from yucky victimy feelings to overeating and numbing out as a way to avoid facing the feelings of victimhood and martyrdom.

The Persecutor

The persecutor is the person or thing that makes the victim feel helpless. If the persecutor is a situation (like your busy schedule), it can feel dominating and oppressive.

However, sometimes we play the role of the persecutor to ourselves. When that happens, the persecutor feels angry, controlling, and judgmental. Maybe you had an overeat and you feel bad. You turn the tables on yourself and transition from the victim to the persecutor.

For example:

- *I should have known better than to think that I could lose weight.*
- *Why did I think I could control myself around birthday party food?*
- *Only a slob would eat the way I do.*
- *I deserve to feel terrible.*

The Rescuer

The rescuer feels satisfaction from helping others and likes to play the hero, to the point of self-sacrificing and neglecting their own needs.

Rescuers like to fix other people's problems and have a need to be needed. (I'm feeling a little uncomfortable right now because I've seen myself in this role more times than I'd like to admit!)

We often do this with our families. We can even take it far enough that we let their needs get in the way of taking care of ourselves. And the whole cycle begins over again.

So how do you get yourself out of this cycle?

1. **When you find yourself playing the role of the victim:**
   First, notice it.
   What kinds of feelings come up? What things do you say that serve as clues that you're in victim mode?
   Next, reclaim your agency.
   You're not helpless. You are powerful!
   Get creative. What are ways to help you feel a small sense of control and take charge of your own situation?
   And thus, the victim becomes the creator.

2. **When you find yourself playing the role of the persecutor:**
   When you find yourself blaming and shaming, stop trying to force and manipulate yourself into change. Accept where you are and that you are doing the best you can. Then ask,
   - *How can I use this experience to motivate me in a positive way?*
   - *What would make me genuinely want to do something different next time?*
   - *What can I do to support myself right now?*
   The persecutor becomes the challenger.

3. **When you find yourself playing the role of the rescuer:**
   Stop solving other people's problems. Empower them to take agency over the things you're doing for them where you can.
   How can you delegate and enable others to take a role in supporting themselves rather than doing it for them?

The rescuer becomes the coach.

Most of this book is about your relationship with yourself. However, it is often the challenges that we have in relationships with others that create worry, stress, and fear that leads to turning to food to numb the pain.

If you find yourself engaging in the victim drama triangle with someone else, try thinking about "The Cosmic Bus Stop" as a way to ease some of the struggle.

The Cosmic Bus Stop

Imagine that before our spirits came to this life in these bodies, we were all at the cosmic bus stop, waiting for the bus to arrive to take us to Earth.

As we're talking to the other souls, we talk about the things we want to learn as souls and spiritual beings. One soul says, "I'm going to learn about grace." Maybe another says, "I want to learn how to forgive."

We need other souls to help us in this Earthly journey to learn the things we set out for ourselves.

What looks like conflict in this Earthly life is actually the gift of love from another soul who agreed to help us in our mission here. It all comes from love and helping us evolve into our higher selves.

I wonder if you and the person you're in relationship with, agreed as souls to come to this life together and help each other learn and grow because your souls love each other so much that you were willing to take on a tough assignment together.

Just a thought!

TOOL #13
How To Get Better Sleep

Stress and sleep have a huge impact on weight loss. When you're stressed, the body responds by pumping cortisol into your body to prepare you to fight or flee.

Cortisol shifts the way you digest food. Because your body is in a stressed state, it moves blood to large muscle groups and away from the digestive system. Therefore, digestion literally slows down and can result in digestive issues as well as a reduced metabolism.

Not so great.

As you probably know, stress can impact sleep. When you're getting less sleep, your brain is tired (obviously).

Because the brain requires a lot of energy from the body, and the brain knows that foods high in sugar, salt, and fat are a quick way to get energy, cravings go up when you're tired.

As mentioned earlier, when you're stressed and tired, blood flow is shunted away from the prefrontal cortex (where you make rational, long-term decisions) to protect the more life sustaining parts of the brain (where you make more impulsive, short-term decisions.)

So when you're tired, your decision-making brain has less blood flow. That makes it extra hard to make good decisions! As you can imagine, that's gonna impact your weight loss efforts over time.

So getting good sleep is a really big deal.

Yet sometimes that's easier said than done.

First, do what you can to set yourself up for successful sleep. Consider your sleep environment.

- Make sure it's dark and cool.
- Keep electronics out of the bedroom.
- Some people do well with white noise.
- Mattress, pillow, and sheet quality make a big difference.
- Use blue light blocking glasses an hour before bed.

Have a pre-sleep routine. Babies aren't the only ones that do well with a predictable nighttime routine.

- Try to go to bed around the same time each night.
- Turn off electronics 30-60 minutes before sleep.
- Try not to eat too close to bedtime. Ideally, you've been done eating for two to three hours before bed.
- Some people like to do stretching or take a warm bath to help them wind down.
- Wear blue light blocking glasses roughly one hour before going to bed to let your brain begin producing melatonin.
- If you need a little extra help getting to sleep, both magnesium and melatonin have been recommended as a sleep supplement.

I don't know about you, but I struggle with waking up in the middle of the night. Falling asleep is usually pretty easy. Staying asleep is a different story.

There always seems to be something available to worry about or ruminate over in the middle of the night. For some reason, the voice in my head is the most negative, the most pessimistic, the most Debbie Downer at 3 a.m.

I've become so familiar with it that I started calling it "The 3 a.m. Voice". So when I wake up in the night and start worrying about something, I'm (usually) able to stop and think *Oh hello 3 a.m. Voice. I've been expecting you. I'm deciding to ignore you right now.*

How would you feel about trying to treat your thoughts in the night as if you were having a conversation with another person? Have you ever seen that Disney movie *Inside Out*? It's sorta like that. Imagine that the voice in your head in the middle of the night is like one of the characters in the movie.

Some folks find that when they can't sleep, a helpful practice can be to get out of bed and meditate for about twenty minutes. I know when I do this, it's amazing the change that happens around minute eighteen. My mind is everywhere for the whole time and then suddenly, I am able to let go and relax and feel ready to go back to bed.

If you find that your mind is racing and meditation is not your thing, just doing a brain dump of all the thoughts to get them out of your head and onto paper can be useful.

TOOL #14
How To Handle the Holidays

"*It's the most wonderful time ❦ of the year.*"
Well, sort of.

The holidays can be a beautiful time to celebrate, reflect, and be together with loved ones. And it can be a time full of stress, anxiety, overwhelm, not-so-holiday-cheer.

There are LOTS of reasons to eat and lots of holiday foods available. It can be a recipe for disaster for your waistline.

Sometimes it feels like once Halloween rolls around, it's downhill from there until January first.

Leftover Halloween candy, Thanksgiving, holiday events and get togethers, cookie exchanges, end of the year parties, college football bowl season, special family holidays, New Years, travel, kids off from school, mother-in-law comes to visit, throw in an anniversary or a birthday and….is it any wonder we gain weight during the holidays?

There's so much going on that it's easy to just throw your hands in the air and say *"Screw it. I'll get back on track once the holidays are over."*

However, from Halloween to January first is about twenty percent of the year. That's no small amount of time!

- What would happen if you decided to just mail it in for twenty percent of your job?

YOU ARE A MIRACLE

- What if you decided to be faithful to your spouse, except for about twenty percent of the time?

You can't give up on twenty percent of anything and expect to succeed.

The holidays don't have to be a disaster and you don't have to be miserable eating lettuce all day either.

With just a little bit of planning and thinking ahead, you'll be amazed at how good you can feel on January first and set yourself up for feeling great in the new year.

How Are You Thinking About It?

A lot of times, we give up before we start. We tell ourselves, *"I can't lose weight during the holidays. There's just too much going on."*

Let's explore that.

1. Make a list of the sentences you're telling yourself about food and healthy habits over the holidays.
2. Write all the reasons why it's hard or why you can't lose weight over the holidays.
3. Ask yourself *"Is this true? What is evidence that the opposite might be true?"*

Example:

1. SENTENCE:
   a. *"I can't lose weight during the holidays."*
2. REASONS:
   a. It's too hard to keep up with everything.
   b. I'm so busy with work and holiday shopping.
   c. There are a lot of holiday events to attend.
   d. I'm super stressed.

338

e. The kids will want to bake cookies.

3. Is this true? What is evidence that the opposite might be true?

   a. It's too hard to keep up with everything.
      i. TRUE?
         • It's true if you tell yourself it is. That becomes a self-fulfilling prophecy. Be careful what you tell yourself. You just might believe it.
      ii. EVIDENCE OF THE OPPOSITE:
         • Are you currently keeping up with things? What are things that don't HAVE to get done right now? When were times in the past that you kept up with things?

   b. I'm so busy with work and holiday shopping.
      i. TRUE?
         • Yeah, it's probably true that you're busy. However, sometimes being busy means we are even more efficient with our time. How can you get more done in smaller chunks of time?
      ii. EVIDENCE OF THE OPPOSITE:
         • What are times of the day or week when you're less busy? Who is someone in your home that is less busy? How can you delegate shopping to those times of the week or to someone else with more time available?

   c. There are a lot of holiday events to attend.

    i. TRUE?

- Probably true. But let's count them up. Exactly HOW MANY events do you have? Three? Five? Fifteen? Getting clear and realistic about the actual number can make you feel a little more control over those events.

    ii. EVIDENCE OF THE OPPOSITE:

- Try this:
  Count up the number of meals you have in a week. Usually that's twenty-one (three meals a day * seven days.) Of those twenty-one meals, how many will be at a holiday event? Probably not more than two or three in a week. That leaves roughly eighteen to nineteen meals of the week that are completely within your control.

d. I'm super stressed.

    i. TRUE?

- Possibly. How might your thoughts be contributing to your feelings of stress? What are you afraid of? What's the worst that could happen if things don't work out perfectly?

    ii. EVIDENCE OF THE OPPOSITE:

- What are things you feel grateful about? What makes you feel relaxed and happy about this time of year?

e. The kids will want to bake cookies.

    i. TRUE?

- Maybe. Have you asked them?
  ii. EVIDENCE OF THE OPPOSITE:
- Maybe there's something else you can create together this year. Maybe do a craft instead of baking things.

Claim your agency.

Sure, there will always be things outside of your control. And if you take time to look at all the things that ARE within your control, there are a lot of things that you could look at differently.

Whatever you're looking for, you'll find it. Look for the things you WANT to find.

Create a Holiday That Is On YOUR Terms

It's easy to worry about what needs to happen to make your mother happy or how to keep Uncle Eddie from getting drunk and insulting your father-in-law.

At the same time, you get to decide what is most important to you. This is a special time of year. What are your favorite things?

Decide what you want from this holiday season.

Notice what the day is about.

Decide what you're gonna care about and what you're not.

It's easy to get wrapped up in the emotional surprises (or just the stress) of the season and eat as a way to soothe over those emotions. But maybe not everything is worth eating over.

Decide what's worth eating emotionally over and what's not.

YOU ARE A MIRACLE

Holiday Anxiety

Let's get really clear on what's going on in your mind.

What are you worried about?

Write it out.

- Whose feelings are you trying not to hurt?
- What family dynamics are you worried about?
- Who drives you crazy that you know will be there?
- What logistics are too tight or too convoluted and make you anxious?
- What if you overeat? How will you treat yourself?

Get it all out on paper.

It's a lot easier to deal with worries when you can see them in the light of day rather than letting them rattle around and have free rein in your brain.

Be Intentional

1. Create a plan. I cannot stress enough how valuable it is to plan ahead.

   You can plan by the day, by the week, or just loosely for the unusual holiday treats that are more available during this time of year.

   Set realistic goals and create a plan to implement them. Do not expect perfection. Make sure your goals and your plans for yourself are realistic and account for travel, fatigue, or unexpected things that come up.

Make your goals super attainable to help yourself feel successful during the season. Little successes help you feel motivated to keep going.

2. Give yourself micro-rewards for following through on your plan. This isn't about saving up for a massage in three weeks. These are mini-high fives you give yourself in the moment when you leave a little bit of wine in the glass and decide that you're done or when you avoid getting seconds of grandma's turkey stuffing.

   It is imperative to give your brain a reason to like following through on your goals so that it will remember to want to keep doing that!

3. What are the treats that just make the season for you? Great! Identify them and plan when you'll have them. How many would make you feel satisfied and not like you overdid it? Decide what's worth splurging over and what's not.

   Make the food earn its way in.

   Give yourself the freedom to splurge. It's okay! Just plan for your splurges versus reacting to the moment.

4. Ask yourself "How do you want to feel on January first?" How can you work backward from that feeling and reverse engineer it to make that a reality?

   Have awareness.

   Don't tune out by telling yourself it's just too hard to lose weight during the holidays. Give yourself the gift of being present with your choices and enjoy everything you choose to put in your mouth.

5. Be prepared to say no. Have a go-to excuse for why you're not eating Aunt Mae's fruit casserole.

   You can decide to share that you're watching what you eat, but sometimes that gets pushed back. If you don't want the comments or the feeling of judgment, try making a joke like "I'm trying to quit." Or "No thanks. I'm driving."

Holiday Tactics

Ok, now let's talk about specific actions you can take to help make this the healthiest holiday season you've ever seen!

Food

1. Don't arrive hungry.
   a. Depriving yourself or restricting your food earlier in the day only makes your brain more freaked out and wanting ALL THE FOOD. Allow yourself to eat sensibly earlier in the day so that you don't arrive at the party starving.
2. Avoid the snack table.
   a. It's easy to lose track of how much you've had when the snacks are small and there's little evidence to show you how much you ate.
   b. If you really want to snack, put it on a plate and portion it out. Decide how much and have that but not more. Try and keep evidence of how much you've had. For example: collect toothpicks from all the pigs-n-blankets so you can see how many you had.

3. Put all snacks and "nibbles" on a plate.
    a. When you're cooking, it can be tempting to just have a "nibble." In the same way that snacks are hard to keep track of, nibbles while you're cooking can add up to a lot more than you think.
    b. Portion out the nibbles you want to have on a plate so that you can see the total amount you want to eat. Have awareness around how much you're eating.
4. Bring your own.
    a. Control the controllables by bringing a healthy dish so you know there's at least something you can fill your plate with. Bringing a veggie tray is an easy go-to.
5. Use smaller plates.
    a. Smaller plates trick your brain into thinking that you ate more. The opposite is also true. Crazy but true.
6. Leave "white space" on your plate.
    a. When serving yourself, try and see the plate beneath your food. If there's so much food on your plate that you can't see the white of the plate underneath it, put a little back.
       You likely won't miss it. And you can always go back if you do.
7. Fill up on healthy foods first.
    a. Look at all the food and try to identify the healthiest thing. Put that on your plate first.
    b. Make the healthier items the bigger portions on your plate.

    c. If you're still hungry, you can always go back. But give yourself a chance to fill up on healthy stuff and just a single serving of the less than healthy things.

8. Avoid or minimize salt and carbs.

    a. Both salty foods and starchy carbs (like pasta, bread, potatoes, and rice) hold water in the body and lead to bloat. If you can avoid these, definitely try. You probably won't miss that extra serving of bread or rolls.

9. Enjoy every bite. Be present.

    a. This food is special! Be there for it. Taste it. Smell it. Chew it. Experience it.

10. Choose your treats and enjoy! Just be intentional about it.

    a. Plan for when you'll eat them and how much. Then enjoy the heck out of those foods! Just plan it versus eating mindlessly.

11. Portion it and freeze the rest.

    a. Leftovers can sit there in your fridge, and you feel like you "should" eat them because you don't want food to go to waste.

    b. If you don't want to toss it, freeze it. Freeze it in single serving sizes so you can thaw one portion at a time.

Exercise

1. Have realistic expectations.

    a. Be imperfect. Any movement, no matter how little or how slow, is still better than sitting on the couch.

    b.   If it's cold out, how can you get in a little movement inside? Walk the stairs, do a YouTube video, play Twister!

2.   Plan a walk.

    a.   Get outside if you can to get Vitamin D and fresh air. Even a short walk to the mailbox and back can help.

3.   Enlist the family.

    a.   What can you do to involve other people? Sometimes if someone else is expecting you to exercise with them, it can make it easier to show up and get moving!

Water

Hydrate all day.

Remember all the ways that water helps you lose weight? Yep, that still counts during the holidays. Plus, it's easy to lose track of how much you drink when you're off of your routine, as we often are during the holidays.

Make a point to drink as much water as you can. It works!

(Also check out the section on How To Drink More Water and Why.)

Alcohol

1.   Sugary drinks add a LOT of calories.

    a.   Things like margaritas, mixers, or eggnog have lots of sugar.

    b.   Try sticking with wine or beer, or a low carb mixed drink like vodka tonic.

2. Go one for one.
    a. Have one glass of water for every drink.
3. Have a cut off.
    a. Identify a cut-off time for when you'll stop drinking.
    b. Identify how many you'd like to have and how many is too many.
4. Plan it.
    a. Just like with your food, be intentional with alcohol. Have a plan ahead of time.

Sleep

1. Less sleep means you're prone to eat more.
2. Prioritize your Zzzzzs to be more in control of your decisions.
3. Get to bed at a regular time.
4. If you're out late, naps are your friend.
5. Cut off caffeine early in the day.
6. Go easy on the booze. Alcohol helps you fall asleep but wrecks the quality of sleep.
   (For more, check out the section on How To Get More Sleep.)

The Aftermath

1. Make a meal plan NOW for the week after the holiday. Create a grocery list too.
2. Plan in some healthy, lighter meals for the days in between holidays and after the holiday.
3. Make it easy on yourself by removing decision fatigue.

4. Plan it now while you have more energy because you'll be tired after the holiday.

TOOL #15
How To Handle Travel

When folks ask me how to help them prepare for travel, I recommend keeping it simple. There's enough going on with travel that you don't need to over-complicate it.

I usually say you only have to remember three things:

1. Drink water
2. Eat a salad every day
3. Move intentionally

If you can manage that, then you'll be okay.

If you want to throw a bonus tip in there, I'd say try to get the best sleep you can.

I don't know about you, but sometimes I can be an anxious traveler. Whether I'm trying to catch a flight or driving for a few hours, my body just seems to know that things are different.

That stress gets translated through my nervous system and into my digestive system. The body knows that when stress comes along, digestion is a less crucial function.

Basically, what that means is it can be four or five days after I get home from travel before my system feels back to normal and "flushed out" from the slower digestion and possibly eating different foods while I was away.

So if you find that the scale isn't saying what you want it to for a few days after you get home, don't sweat it. It's normal for your body to need a few days to get back to "all systems go."

CONCLUSION
YOU ARE A MIRACLE

THE GOLDEN BUDDHA
(Psst, even if you skip other parts, be sure to read this!)

In 1957, workers at a monastery in Thailand were moving a giant clay statue of the Buddha when ropes broke, and the statue fell hard on the ground.

When one of the monks inspected the statue, he noticed a golden light emanating from between the cracks in the clay. Using a hammer and chisel to chip away at the clay, the monk realized that the statue was actually made entirely of solid gold underneath.[35,36]

Historians surmise that the statue was created nearly 700 years ago. In the eighteenth century, the Ayutthaya kingdom was under siege by Burmese invaders who were known for melting the gold of the nations they conquered.

It is believed that monks plastered over the golden nature of the Budda in 1767 to prevent it from being stolen and melted by the Burmese invaders. Eventually the monastery was destroyed

---

35 https://www.windstarcruises.com/blog/history-of-thailands-golden-buddha/
36 https://carolyntate.co/the-story-of-the-golden-buddha/

by the raiders and the statue lay among the ruins without attracting much attention.

Over the years, the statue was moved to various locations, and its true nature was forgotten for nearly 200 years.

Until a crack in the outer mud revealed the beauty beneath.

Just like the Golden Buddha, you already have that light within you.

Many of my clients just want to feel confident and to be able to love themselves for who they are. The truth is, that love and worthiness is already inside you, and it is closer than you think.

You were born as a spiritual being into this human body. You came out of the womb fascinated by your fingers and toes and the amazing things that your body could do. You knew you were worthy simply by existing.

However, as you grew and internalized messages from your environment, you added layer upon layer of clay and mud over the Golden Buddha within yourself. But instead of mud, you used limiting stories and negative beliefs to cover up your light. Eventually, you became so covered in clay that you forgot the true beauty and magnificence of who you are underneath.

The key to rediscovering your own Golden Buddha and genuinely loving yourself is to first realize that what you seek is already within you. Your work is to gradually chip away at the clay of limiting stories and limiting beliefs from the outside world. Little by little, as you let go of those heavy stories, you begin to let your inner light shine.

*"Remember: You have a light within you, the Holy Spirit.
And wherever you go you will bring a light greater than
the darkness around you."*
Bear Gryllis

How can you look for the light within you today by examining and chipping away at a limiting story that might be covering up your innate magnificence?

YOU HAVE A GIFT WORTH GIVING.

Don't wait.

Don't sleep on your dream.

The world needs what only you can give us.

Don't keep waiting to live your life until that moment when you finally lose the weight and feel like you can do the things you want to do.

Do them now.

Live now.

Be 100% fully, gorgeously you, now.

You deserve it.

Remind yourself every day, *"I have a gift worth giving. My voice was meant to be heard. This life is a gift and it's meant for living, not waiting. And I choose to be all 100% imperfectly me today."*

Don't wait.

We're counting on you.

You Are a Miracle.

RESOURCES

If you're interested in learning more from books on psychology, the brain, and beliefs, you might enjoy any of the following:

Atomic Habits by James Clear (Avery)

Breaking the Habit of Being Yourself by Joe Dispenza (Hay House)

Dark Horse by Todd Rose (Harper One)

How To Be An Imperfectionist by Stephen Guise (Selective Entertainment LLC)

How To Fail At Almost Everything And Still Win Big by Scott Adams (Portfolio)

Learned Optimism by Martin Seligman (Alfred A. Knopf)

Mindset by Carol Dweck (Random House)

One Small Step can Change Your Life: The Kaizen Way by Robert Mauer (Workman Publishing Company)

Personality Isn't Permanent by Benjamin Hardy (Portfolio)

Psycho-Cybernetics by Maxwell Maltz (TarcherPerigee)

Self-Compassion by Kristin Neff (Harper-Collins)

Smarter, Better, Faster by Charles Duhigg (Random House)

Soundtracks by Jon Acuff (Baker Books)

The Alter Ego Effect by Todd Herman (Harper Business)

The Compound Effect by Darren Hardy (Hachette Go)

The Gifts of Imperfection by Brene Brown (Random House)

The Happiness Advantage by Shawn Achor (Currency)

The Magic of Thinking Big by David Schwartz (Prentice Hall Press)

The Progress Principle by Teresa Amiable (Harvard Business Review Press)

The Willpower Instinct by Kelly McGonigal (Avery)

Whole Brain Living by Jill Bolte Taylor (Hay House Inc)

Women, Food, and God by Geneen Roth (Scribner)

You Are A Badass by Jen Sincero (Running Press Adult)

ACKNOWLEDGEMENTS

This book would not be a reality without the love and support of so many people.

Thank you to my husband Steve, for so many things. For believing in me when I didn't. For being my sounding board, my confidant, and my greatest cheerleader when I needed it most. You used to say that fifty-one percent of your success was due to me. Well, more than fifty-one percent of my success is due to you because you believe in me. Thank you.

To Robby and Annie, thank you for your support and un-wavering knowledge that "Of course you're going to publish your book...because that's what heroes do." You gave me the gift of seeing myself through your eyes. You helped me more than you know and you lift me up every day. Thank you.

Thank you to my parents, Mike and Donna Born, for al-ways loving me, supporting me, and believing that I am capable of anything. I could thank you every day and it would not begin to cover it.

Thank you to Theresa and David Merritt for always asking me how the book was coming and expressing your stalwart faith in me.

The most sincere thank you to Kelli Watson. My friend, my coach, my colleague, my publisher. Without you, I would not have realized my calling as a coach. And I most certainly would not have crossed the finished line with this book. Thank you for so many gr8t gifts you've given me!

To Jesse Martini for our coaching sessions. You helped me through our conversations and by believing in me. You were pivotal in helping me get started. Thank you.

Thank you to Susie Rolander for always cheering me on and for giving me the feedback that my work is worth sharing.

To Bob Thompson. Thank you for all our many wonderful and thought provoking conversations.

To my dear friends, Christy Kern, Tree Branch, Gena Ferrabee, Christy Sharafinski, Dori Zabari, and Summer Howard. Thank you for supporting me.

Thank you to Lynn Waidelich for asking me to join your Stroller Strides group, where it all began. You helped set me on a path I didn't even know was there. Thank you.

To my clients, past, present, and future. Every day you give me the gift of letting me help you look in the mirror and see yourself for the miracle you already are. Thank you.

Confident Body Coach
THE HEART + SCIENCE OF WEIGHT LOSS

Looking for support implementing these ideas and making sustainable change a reality in your life?

It's one thing to know information intellectually. It's another thing to put it into action in real life when you've got a busy schedule and kid's snacks in the pantry are just calling your name at 3:42pm on a Tuesday.

If you'd like to learn more about how to work one on one with me please visit:
https://confidentbody.coach/private-coaching

I'd love to meet you!

Confident Body Coach
THE HEART + SCIENCE OF WEIGHT LOSS

Made in the USA
Monee, IL
25 April 2024